JOURNEY
through the
STORM

*a faith walk
through
cancer*

SUZANNE TUCKER

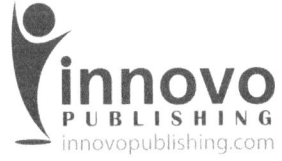

innovo
PUBLISHING
innovopublishing.com

Innovo Publishing
159 College Street
Collierville, TN 38017
www.innovopublishing.com
888-546-2111

Providing full-service Christian publishing for authors, artists and ministries.
Books, eBooks, Audiobooks, Music & Film.

ISBN: 978-1-61314-357-5
Library of Congress: 2012936457

Table of Contents

Acknowledgements

To the Lord, Jesus Christ, whose Presence makes all the difference in every situation in life. The journey shared in this book is a testimony to His amazing and loving grace, His power and His faithfulness to frail humanity.

To Charlie, my best friend, lover, and faithful husband for 45 years: Thank you for your Godly influence and patience, your constant encouragement, and your persevering love. You are steadfast, and that didn't change during the year of cancer treatment. When I was ready to give up, you gave me the motivation to keep moving forward and to press on to reach the goal. You have challenged me to be the best person I can be and to accomplish far more than I would have dreamed possible. So much of what I know about God is from seeing Him in you. I admire the man you are. I love you more than words can say.

To Carie, thank you for sharing life with me. Your daily encouragement has been unending. Your medical knowledge and presence at my doctor's appointments during that year were invaluable. You knew the right questions and answers when I was overwhelmed with emotions. Your hours of editing have not only greatly improved this journal but have also taught me how to be a better writer and communicator. I watch you persevere in helping other women with breast cancer and believe God is going to use your work in amazing ways. Thank you for being my friend as well as my daughter.

To Christie, who always has an encouraging word, makes life a party, and adds the "delight" to every event: You have brought joy when I was too down or tired to think; you made me laugh. Your encouragement has lifted me more times than I can count. You have helped me so many times get beyond the present situation to see beyond and to look up. Your creativity has helped to give me a different perspective when I felt stuck in a situation, a mindset, or a generational attitude. I love the many things I learn through you and Chris about God's far-reaching love to every person. I thank God for the gift of your and Chris' lives to our family and for your support through this challenging journey.

To Dianna, who has walked with me for years, and prayed faithfully: Your encouragement has always been a precious gift. Thank you for the hours you spent editing and for your insights that have come at just the right time. Your comments in this journal always spoke to me, and I am sure they have impacted the lives of all who read my blog. You are a dear friend and I treasure you, even across the miles.

To Jeri Daniels, I am grateful for your long-time friendship, love and encouragement, as well as your creative giftedness. Thank you for allowing me to use your photograph of the storm. It continues to minister to me as I walk the pathway of daily life.

To Dr. Lynn Canavan, for your understanding and medical insights, your surgical expertise, and your personal care, I thank you.

To Dr. Monte Jones, for your continued care in treating me, in addition to your expertise and wisdom, I am truly grateful. It makes a difference to have doctors you trust. Your entire staff is wonderful. To Holly, you touch lives and diffuse fears with your endless smiles, gentleness, and step-by-step explanations. To Kathy and Kathy, thank you for your continued help and encouragement; you are treasured gifts to this patient.

To each of you, too numerous to list, who have walked with me through life, being a spiritual example and pointing me toward Jesus, I thank you. For every prayer you have prayed for me and my family, I am eternally grateful. Thank you for your patient understanding and support through the year of breast cancer treatment. Every comment written on the CaringBridge journal and every email touched my heart. I wish I could have published each comment in this book. They were a source of life and strength every day. Your continued friendships are a gift from God. Thank you and may the Lord bless you immeasurably.

Preface

Dearest Elisabeth, Rebekah, Cella, Nathaniel, and baby Emmy,

The primary purpose for my publishing this journal is to share with you the testimony of God's amazing faithfulness to me personally, to our family, and even to you. First, I want you to see in these pages that as you walk through challenging, even life-threatening, situations, God is there with you. He will never leave you. He is very near when you walk through trials. He can be trusted with anything and everything in your life.

This does not mean that you will avoid having fears, questions, doubts, or emotional struggles. It does mean that when you do experience those things, you can turn to Him and He will show you how to deal with them. That is part of life with Jesus. He will use the situations of your life to conform you to His character and to build the integrity of His fruit in your life. But for this to happen, you must rely on Him. Study His Word, trust His promises, and fulfill the conditions. That is the way to a fulfilling life here on earth and is preparation for your eternal life in Heaven.

The second message I want to share with you is that you must surrender your life to Him and not try to reason or work things out on your own. You cannot do it alone. You were not meant to live without Him or without the strength of other strong believers. We were not created to be independent, but to wholly depend on Him. Ask Him to surround you with others who believe in Him enough that their character and their actions line up with their words and who will stand with you even in hard times.

Your PawPaw is one of those people. He has not only been a strong support during this challenging journey, but he has been an encourager to me through our 45 years of marriage. He was the one who led me to the Lord, primarily through his example of Godliness. He has been an accountability partner who expected me to live a Godly life. When I fell short, he would take me by the hand and teach me how God wanted me to live. He was willing to speak truth to me, even when I was not sure that I wanted to hear. I am who I am today because of Jesus in my life and because of your grandfather's amazing love and commitment to God and to his family.

And the third thing I want you to know and grasp for yourself is that prayer is essential to the Christian life. Prayer is not talking *to* God. It only begins there. Prayer is a two-way conversation that helps you grow in your personal relationship with Him. As I write this, four of you have asked Jesus into your hearts. That is the beginning of your walk with Him. That is the starting point of your lifelong response to His amazing and pursuing love for you. His desire is for much more. Spend time getting to know Him. He wants a constant relationship with you that involves communication. Always be honest with Him. For you to do that, you must be honest with yourself. Honesty is not always easy, but it is essential. It requires humility on your part and willingness to open your heart. That is what true Christianity is about. It is not a list of rules for you to follow; it is a close, intimate relationship in which you experience the vastness of His love for you.

I hope you will see His love extended to me as I was going through this challenging year. But, our response to His amazing love is to return it to Him, to love Him enough to want to be pleasing to Him in everything we do.

I prayed for each of you before you were born. More importantly, God had you in His heart long before you were born. He created you for a specific and amazing purpose and with a destiny that is far beyond what you can imagine. I pray daily that each of you will find the destiny He has for your life. And I also pray that your love and trust for Him will greatly exceed mine.

I love each of you for who you are. I love God for His creativity in making you with your strengths and weaknesses, gifts and talents, and even the inabilities that He purposed for you. It is in those weaknesses that He will be the strongest. And I love Him for the gift that each of you are to me and to our family.

He is a good Father and will always take care of you, when you walk through good times or hard times. Trust Him, my precious ones. He is trustworthy and faithful beyond our imagination or comprehension.

With so much love,

Grammy

8

$\mathcal{D}$ear Elisabeth, Rebekah, and Nathaniel,

I will never forget Christmas 2007. Mom, your Grammy, grabbed me as she came into the house and said, "I need to show you something." We went into my bedroom, and she showed me the breast mass she had found. I was dumbfounded: we didn't know if the mass was cancerous, but the fear I felt at that moment was sickening. Most of the day, I thought about that mass, silently begging God to make it all go away.

Life is not always predictable. And bad things happen. We don't know why. We just have to trust that God knows all and that when we release our circumstances to Him, He is faithful and is in control of every step of our lives. Through the next eight months, I saw Grammy live with that trust.

I also had to face my own fears. I wasn't terribly afraid that I too would someday have breast cancer or that you, my children, would have to experience that. Perhaps that's because from the very beginning, Grammy and I prayed, separately and together, that God would stop the pattern of cancer in her family and that it would not be a legacy that would be passed on to future generations. I knew God would be faithful and would be Lord of the health of our family. When I had my own irregular mammogram a few months after she was diagnosed with cancer, I immediately called Grammy and asked her to pray. After having a sonogram, we knew the Lord had begun to answer our prayers when the doctor said there was nothing irregular as the radiologist had thought.

My fear concerned life without Grammy. Without her, I would be alone, and I selfishly wasn't ready for that. I wanted her to be here for my graduation and for your graduations, weddings, and children. I wanted her to see all of that, but I also wanted you to have the blessing of grandparents who participated in your lives.

Through the experience, the Lord taught each of us a number of lessons. I learned how to assert myself in personal medical care by asking questions, reading about Grammy's disease, and researching online. I was able to help her with the information I learned. I strengthened my resolve to not compromise the priority of family when work and school demanded a lot. And I learned how to trust God in a deeper way.

God created opportunities for all members of our family to reach out to others. I took y'all to the infusion room and encouraged you to talk to other people and not to fear medical treatments. We visited Grammy during treatments and provided support during the duration of her care. I communicated with and provided meals for several friends who were also battling cancer.

As a result of Grammy's experience, I began to focus my own research on breast cancer. I am researching how, why, and what patients battling breast cancer communicate online. I hope after I write my dissertation to work on publications about privacy, security, and patients' rights. Perhaps my research will help other women to communicate effectively, yet at the same time protect themselves when they share in online communities.

Yes, I'm glad that Mom is healed and the battle with breast cancer is over. And although the experience was frightening and painful, I don't wish that it had never happened because so many good things resulted. No, life is not predictable, but God uses all experiences for our good and His glory.

I love you,

Mom (Carie)

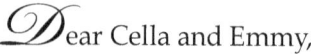ear Cella and Emmy,

Like me, you have been very fortunate to grow up in a Christian home, where the core of what we do, who we are, and how we live are based on the true Word of God. Knowing who God is and how He sees you are truths that will become second nature to you, because we began teaching you those things as infants. But the time will come, as it does in everyone's life, where you will have to genuinely determine if what you claim to believe about God is, in fact, what you believe. Some might say, "Put your money where your mouth is," and prove that your faith and trust in God are more than songs you sing and words you say. Life will bring you to a place where you realize you are not in control. And that's when it becomes your turn to either doubt God's ability to be God or to decide to trust Him in all things.

Sometimes making that decision takes a long time — not necessarily because you lack faith in God, but because the circumstances are so big that they catch you off guard and scare you, or maybe wound you, and you have to reach down into the deepest corners of your heart and search for the faith that was once strong. But sometimes that decision takes an instant. You just know that you are not in the driver's seat, and so you stop trying to grab for the steering wheel. You get out of the way and trust that God is going to be there, never doubting that His plan is good.

When Grammy was diagnosed with cancer, my decision took only an instant. I was incredibly sad that she was suffering and facing the unknown that accompanies the word "cancer." But from the very beginning, I knew that the fear of what *could* happen and what *might* happen was too heavy a burden for me to carry. I knew I couldn't even pick it up, much less carry it during the long journey ahead, so I had to ask God to carry it for me. He did, just as He promises (1 Peter 5:7). My prayer was always that God would heal Grammy, but that in all things He would provide grace and peace to face whatever came our way.

I'm so glad that through this journal you will get a glimpse of what Grammy experienced during this time. You will see how God can use what people call "bad" for His good and His glory. I hope you are reminded that life is fleeting, that your circumstances can change in an instant, and that you should not take one day or one hug or one moment for granted. Above all, I hope you see that God is good all the time, regardless of our circumstances, and He is near to us.

It is because of the Lord's loving-kindness that we are not destroyed for His loving-pity never ends. It is new every morning. He is so very faithful (Lamentations 3:22-23 NLV).

With love,

Mom (Christie)

Author's Note

The pages that follow represent my ongoing journal that I kept from the time of my diagnosis of breast cancer until the days just after I was deemed cancer free.

I regularly posted these comments on CaringBridge.com, a nonprofit website that provides a private venue enabling medical patients to detail their experiences and enables visitors to my site to reply to my posts.

Paragraphs labeled *GUEST* are compiled from some of the online replies (from family and friends as well as from total strangers) I received after my CaringBridge journal entries.

Journey through the Storm
Journal

Wednesday, February 20 — Receiving the Diagnosis

On January 11, after numerous tests and a biopsy, I was diagnosed with breast cancer. The surgeon gave me several options for treatment and her recommendations. Because of the tumor's location, the surgeon could not remove the tumor without a complete mastectomy. She scheduled major surgery for February 15. Then the surgeon took me to the office of an oncologist who talked about possible options for treatment. After receiving test results from the surgery, his recommendation is chemotherapy.

Even though I don't know the details of the future, I determined not to cancel any previous commitments. God, in His sovereignty, has already created opportunities for me to minister, and I trust Him to give me the strength and ability to fulfill those commitments. God is not surprised by what is happening, and I believe that, as He has said in the Bible, He will guide my steps in the months ahead.

Before the diagnosis, I accepted an invitation to speak at a women's conference in Japan in early February, so we scheduled surgery around my trip. My time in Japan was restful. When I was not speaking or fellowshipping with the Japanese ladies, I was in my hotel room resting and preparing for the next session. At the end of the conference, I told the ladies that when I returned home I would undergo cancer surgery, and they gathered around me and prayed for my healing. I returned home emotionally, physically, and spiritually prepared for surgery. The day after I returned to Texas, I had a pre-op appointment and two days later had surgery.

It has been five days since my surgery. The doctor was able to remove the entire 2" tumor with a cancer-free zone around it. There were a few challenges during and after surgery, but I am recovering and grateful to have it behind me.

Thursday, February 21 — Establishing My Crisis Theology

A few years ago, my pastor's wife asked me to begin a ministry at church, spending time with people going through crisis. I sought the Lord for direction for the ministry, but I did not receive an answer for six months. One day, I had lunch with a long-time friend, and as we talked, I realized she was giving vision for the ministry.

She talked about having "crisis theology." I didn't even know what that meant. She explained that we must know how God feels about people in crisis, how He treats them, and what the Scriptures say about crisis situations.

After our meeting, I began to read the Bible with a new focus. I reread the New Testament Gospels—Matthew, Mark, Luke, and John—to see how Jesus treated people who were living through difficult situations. I reread the Old Testament book of Job, and then I went through the Psalms to learn what David had to say *about* and *to* God when he was in a desperate situation. I also read to glean what God said back to David.

God does not turn His back on, condemn, or ignore those who are going through crises. Jesus always ministered to those in pain. He says we will face problems, but He has overcome the world (John 16:33). His love is constant and sustains us, and often He demonstrates that love through other people. Even now, I see how God used this new ministry to prepare me to walk through the upcoming months. David's words in the Psalms continue to encourage me:

> Even though I walk through the valley of the shadow of death, I fear no evil, for You are with me . . . (Psalm 23:4 NASB).

> The cords of Sheol surrounded me; The snares of death confronted me. In my distress I called upon the Lord, And cried to my God for help; He heard my voice out of His temple, And my cry for help before Him came into His ears (Psalm 18:5–6 NASB).

> *I would have despaired* unless I had believed that I would see the goodness of the Lord In the land of the living. Wait for the Lord; Be strong and let your heart take courage; Yes, wait for the Lord (Psalm 27:13–14 NASB).

> You are my hiding place; You preserve me from trouble; You surround me with songs of deliverance (Psalm 32:7 NASB).

> The steps of a man are established by the Lord, And He delights in his way. When he falls, he shall not be hurled headlong, Because the Lord is the One who holds his hand. I have been young, and now I am old, Yet I have not seen the righteous forsaken Or his descendants begging bread (Psalm 37:23–25 NASB).

Today is a good day. My goal has been to do laundry, though Charlie has already done most of it, and to bake an apple pie for dinner! Pretty sweet goals, huh?

Tomorrow morning very early, I must be at the hospital for a heart scan. I don't know what that involves but only that it is important before the next surgery and before I begin chemotherapy. When the nurse called to confirm my appointment, I thanked her for the "early appointment" and jokingly told her that because I don't wake up until 9 a.m., the tests will be finished before I realize I am awake. She said that was a wonderful attitude. I want to have a joyful attitude and leave God's print on each person I meet. I don't want people to remember me, but I desire that they have an encounter with God and His love.

As I have read and reread the precious notes from each of you, I have cried. Thank you for your ministry to me. Your love and encouragement are not just words but LIFE — and I can feel it inside, building me up. Your words have brought joy and strength to me today. What a gift.

I hurt for those who walk this path alone. My prayer today is for them. May the Lord guide their paths to some of you, so they too may receive your life-giving encouragement. Also, today I am thanking God for you and your impact on my life and my family.

❧ GUEST

I've been reading Philip Yancey's book *Prayer: Does It Make Any Difference?*[1] and this morning read his quote of Dr. Paul Brand:

> A person experiences maximum health when body, soul, and spirit are aligned in a way that expresses the will of the Designer. Those who pray for the sick and suffering should first praise God for the remarkable agents of healing designed into the body, and then ask that God's special grace give the suffering person the ability to use those resources to their fullest advantage. I have seen remarkable instances of physical healing accomplished in this way. The

prayers of fellow Christians can offer real, tangible help by setting into motion the intrinsic powers of healing in a person controlled by God. This approach does not contradict natural laws; rather, it fully employs the design features built into the human body (p. 254).

Yancey concludes by saying,

A person who is at peace, surrounded by loving support, will quite literally heal better, drawing on the resources of body, mind, and spirit. Such healing is not inferior to direct intervention by God that reverses physical laws. Rather, the Spirit uses the natural milieu—the mind, nerves, and hormonal systems that govern all cells—to accomplish the work (p. 254).

I love you,
Glenda

Saturday, February 23 — Experiencing Daily Miracles

Your prayers are one of the most valuable gifts you give me. I know that God hears and answers prayers, although I also know He doesn't always answer them as we might want or expect.

This week a friend called and asked how I was doing. When I told her the treatment the doctors have recommended, she said God had already told her. I was comforted to hear what she had to say. I know that God can heal me instantly, and I am very grateful that people have prayed for that healing. However, I have heard Him say that I will walk through the "process of healing." My friend confirmed that God had told her the same thing.

Several people have said to me, "I don't want you to have to go through this!" Their caring blesses me. However, I began to think about how God loves His children and how He has carefully chosen my path to healing. If I could see all that God is doing and will do in and through me in the next six months, I might choose this difficult path rather than avoid it. I do know that He must work this for my good and for His glory, as He has already committed in His Word (Romans 8:28). I can hardly wait to see how that comes about.

I said something about not receiving the "miracle healing" and my friend's response was that God told her I will see miracles! In fact, she said that I will see miracles daily — that He will give me months of miracles, and that those miracles will come in many forms. I will have pain and it will instantly lift, and that will be a miracle. At times, the doctors will predict certain side effects, and I won't have them, and that will be a miracle. She also said that peoples' lives will be touched and changed through my experience, and that will be a miracle.

I have often asked God to take the situations of my life and use them to minister to the lives of others. He is answering that prayer.

Many of you have prayed for a miracle in my life. The Lord has assured me that He will work a miracle for every time one of you has asked Him to do so. One Sunday in church, more than 100 people prayed that I would be healed. That must be worth a couple of months of miracles! I thank you again for all the prayers. I promise to share as I see the miracles happen.

Thank you again for all the precious notes. I can already tell that checking this website is going to be a highlight of each day. Your words encourage and strengthen me.

And by the way, we did get the pie made and it was wonderful! Yes, Keri, it was the sugar-free pie recipe! Yum! :-)

Sugar Free Apple Pie
(adapted from a recipe in a military wives' cookbook[2])

Preheat oven to 350 degrees. Place unbaked piecrust in pie plate.

Peel, core, and slice 6–8 large apples. Place in the piecrust. (I often substitute peaches, plums, pears, or a combination of fruits instead of apples and add Craisins®, grapes, or berries.)

Empty 1 12-oz. can frozen concentrated apple or white grape juice into saucepan; bring to a boil.

Add ¼ cup cold water, mixed with 3 tablespoons cornstarch and 1 teaspoon cinnamon. Continue to boil, stirring constantly until mixture thickens. Pour thickened juice over fruit.

With second piecrust, make lattice topping. (Lattice topping, rather than a solid pie crust, allows the steam to escape and fruit is crunchy rather than mushy.)

Bake at 350 degrees for 45–60 minutes, until brown.

❧ *GUEST*

I am delighted, amazed, and blessed at the response to your website. You still receive the blessing of encouragement from these saints, and you can focus not on the disease but on God's love through these dear ones!

Someone said today, "You have my sympathy about your mother." I had to smile, and I answered her: "Thank you, but I think my mom considers this a calling. Every time she goes to the hospital, she finds someone who needs God's touch, and she stops and prays for that person." The irony is that you wouldn't have this opportunity if it weren't for your circumstances.

I am so proud of you, my beloved mother and friend.

Carie

❧ *GUEST*

I read this verse this morning and you came to mind: "You are my hiding place; you will protect me from trouble and surround me with songs of deliverance" (Psalm 32:7).

This is exactly what God is doing in your life. Bless you, my dear friend. I also pray strength, comfort, and peace for your family as they walk with you. Keep setting those sweet goals and keep shining for Jesus!

Much love,
Lissa

❧ *GUEST*

This morning, as I was praying for you, the Lord brought to mind Psalm 23:4-6 —

Even though I walk through the valley of the shadow of death, I will fear no evil, for *you are with me* [emphasis added]; your rod and your staff, they comfort me. You prepare a table before me in the presence of my enemies. You anoint my head with oil; my cup overflows. Surely goodness and love will follow me all the days of my life, and I will dwell in the house of the Lord forever.

I hear the Lord assuring me that your ministry will not be limited by this season in your life — that just as a field is allowed to rest during the seventh year, you are being allowed to rest. And what comes after the rest is JUBILEE! This morning I prayed that you would not experience any side effects from the chemotherapy. Then I read your journal from 02/23 — God is definitely mobilizing the army!

> I love you!
> Linda

❧ GUEST

Right now, we are praying for and with a wonderful neighbor who has been diagnosed with brain cancer. . . . I have asked if I can read to her and she has said, "Yes." What a delight to give in any way I can to bring light, truth, and blessing. God is dealing with me about what worship really is and I see it as obeying the Holy Spirit even as Jesus is our example. It is certainly more than a song.

> Love,
> Darleen

❧ GUEST

Cella tried to post last night, but we had technical issues. She wrote out her note so I could try again on her behalf.

"Hi, Grammy. I love you. I have been praying for you all day. I think you are lovely and I like all the food you make. It was fun to see you and PawPaw last night. You are both so silly." Love, Cella

The kids learned about Daniel in the lions' den last night at Life Group. As I prepared the lesson for them, God was reminding me that His power wasn't shown by keeping Daniel out of the den. The testimony came from Daniel going into the den and coming out unharmed. God doesn't promise to keep us out of the scary dens of life, but He does give the angels charge over us while we are there.

> Love you, Mom!
> Christie

I know that Carie has mentioned me to you as one who has traveled this road for the past year. She has been such a blessing time and again by bringing meals and helping with kids.

I now look forward to the privilege of encouraging you and others who face this monster head-on. I will certainly pray for you and I want you to feel free to email or call me anytime you need to pick the brain of someone who has been there. So many wonderful women came forward during my treatment and gave encouragement, not to mention lots of great tips, and I want to do the same.

Susan

Tuesday, February 26 — Experiencing the Power of Kind Words

Yesterday, I had a follow-up appointment after surgery. The surgeon says I am doing well, and she took out the drain. I am *drain free*! YEAH! This may not sound like a big reason to celebrate, but it means that now I can take a shower. That *is* worth celebrating. I have taken much for granted in life and am becoming more aware of and grateful for small things.

March 7 is the date of my next surgery. I am thankful to have time to begin to recover from the first surgery before having the rest of the work done.

It may sound strange, but I look forward to each trip to the hospital. Every time I go, I see people who are alone and hurting. Often, I want to walk over and hug them. Sometimes I do.

Yesterday, when Charlie and I were at the hospital, I watched him minister to two elderly women. Both were obviously very sick. One was alone and had on a wig. As we walked by, he told her how beautiful she was. I watched her eyes go from a dull sadness to a bright sparkle after he spoke. She lifted her head and straightened her back. A big smile came across her face that replaced the sad and weary look that had been there. It was so precious.

Later, as we were sitting in the surgeon's waiting room, another lady came out of the doctor's office. She looked to be in her middle 80s and was having a very difficult time walking with her walker. Charlie said hello to her as he jumped up to open the door for her. Then he told her that she looked like a million dollars and that her silver hair was beautiful. Where she had been dragging her feet and having a hard time walking, there came a quickness to her step. And again, I saw the sparkle light up in her eyes. I got a glimpse of a beautiful young woman residing inside of her. Such little things like a kind word make a big difference.

Charlie always has a kind word to say to those he meets. I learn much about God's love by watching the way he cares about people.

Often, we think "witnessing" is preaching the Gospel and giving people Scriptures. There is a time for that and it is valuable. But I have seen Charlie impact lives with a simple word of kindness. I have seen the smiles and the sparkle come to their eyes, sometimes just because he acknowledges them and asks how they are doing. He goes out of his way to talk to and praise veterans. And like those ladies, he knows who needs a compliment.

It should not be difficult to touch lives. I have been thinking that if I will be more aware of others than of myself and will determine to love everyone I meet, I can also reach out to people and bring joy into their lives, even in simple ways.

If I were not walking through this situation, we would not be in the hospital and these lives might not be touched. God is graciously providing opportunities for us, and today I am very thankful for the way He redeems all situations in our lives and uses them for our good and for His glory. Before this situation arose, a lady at church spoke to me saying that a whirlwind was coming into my life that would take me out of my comfort zone and move me to the place where God needed me to be. I had no idea that the hospital would be where He would need me to go and minister. I desire to use every opportunity possible to touch other hurting people with God's love.

Thank you again for your encouragement and prayers. You may never know on this earth the difference your words make in my life.

⋙ GUEST

Thank you for sharing about Charlie's ministry of compliments! How precious — it acknowledges the soul and sees the beauty that God sees as well as the potential. That speaks deeply to me.

I appreciate your heart to press into a path with God that allows others to see His grace and abundance as you are squeezed and weakened.

We trust our Lord with you for the glory that comes from faithfulness in suffering, the wisdom of patient endurance, and the sustaining grace to bring forth fruit one hundred-fold. Though our own paths vary, I believe many are walking with you toward the goal of God's destiny through this.

Dianna

GUEST

Mrs. Tucker,

As I get older, it starts to seem silly to me that I still call you that, but it is who you have always been to me. When I was little, you were the Mrs. Tucker who taught me the piano and made my beautiful pink princess cake with a real Barbie in the middle. You were also the Mrs. Tucker that I knew would take care of me and all four brothers and sisters if anything ever happened to my parents. (My parents have probably never been covered in prayer as much as they were then!)

In college, you were the Mrs. Tucker who welcomed me into your home when I was desperately homesick and gave me a home away from home and baked wonderful apple pies without sugar! I was always amazed at how good it was! Then you were the Mrs. Tucker who was an intricate part of my wedding, as your whole family was.

I still have the quilt that you made out of all the cross-stitch squares that my friends made for my first baby. Every time my boys see it, I tell them about Mrs. Tucker and how every stitch in that blanket represents prayers on their behalf.

Now, you are the Mrs. Tucker that I consider a spiritual mentor. The long conversations filled with laughter and tears and prayer and tons of encouragement that we have had over Mexican food. The Mrs. Tucker that still sends me cards and emails that are so humbling to me and yet so full of love. The Mrs. Tucker who has taken both of my sisters under her wing.

I find myself so amazed at how you are coping with everything. I just want to be like you. Please know that you are very loved and that in my simpleness, I will be praying desperately on your behalf. Like I told you before, Satan obviously does not know who he is messing with!

I love you!
Keri

Thursday, February 28 — Celebrating This Year

Charlie and I have made a decision — we will not put the Christmas tree away. After the holidays, other things took priority, and then I didn't have time or energy to take down the tree. When I came home from the hospital, we both admitted that the tree, covered with "crismons" (Christian symbols) is an encouragement to us. This Christmas, even more than ever before, we celebrated Christ, the Prince of Peace, as the sole source of our hope.

Every year since 1978, the Lord has given us a word of guidance for the coming year. This year, we had not received a word. We wondered if the Lord was doing something different. However, on January 9, Charlie was working in the garden, preparing it for planting. As he worked, the Lord said, "You and Suzanne will *celebrate* all year" — the word we had been waiting and listening for. What amazing timing, which is so like the Lord. Only two days later, I was diagnosed with cancer.

Some would think that word is not compatible with our circumstances, but it was God's instruction for how I am to walk through the events of the coming year.

After seeing the doctor and being told I had cancer, we left the hospital and went to some friends' home for dinner. When we walked in, the wife said, "I hope you don't mind. The Lord told us that this evening would be a celebration!" They had no idea what God had spoken to us or what the doctor had said. After sharing the information we received from the doctor, we focused on the word God had spoken to us and confirmed through them. We had a wonderful dinner and celebrated.

Charlie and I rejoice in the gift of His Word to prepare us for this journey. The Lord has continued to reveal to us some of the exciting things we will celebrate this year. But we have found that the blessings of life and relationships (you) are reasons to celebrate each day.

My children are probably laughing. I have said for years that someday I would find a way to leave the tree up all year. I didn't expect that to happen before I was about 98 years old. But this is the year. It will stay up, at least until late next summer when cancer treatment is complete. In the meantime, we continue to rejoice in His presence in our lives, and enjoy the tree . . . but with the shutters closed!

✂ GUEST

Yes, I'm laughing, but with joy, because leaving the tree up shows me that we don't need to fear your circumstances — we can celebrate life together. Isn't that what Christmas is about: celebrating Jesus' life and the life that we gain because of Him?

Love you both so much!
Carie

✂ GUEST

Almost from the very moment that Carie told me about what you are facing, God impressed upon me that this would be a time of rejoicing and for Him to be glorified. Your updates and various comments on this site are a testament to that — God is not just great, He is very good too.

I hope your Christmas tree is artificial.

Bill

✂ GUEST

We continue to pray recovery, healing, and protection for Suzanne. We believe grace and peace will be multiplied unto you! We love you so much! Shalom!

Bless the Lord, O my soul: And all that is within me, bless His holy name. Bless the Lord, O my soul, And forget not all His benefits: Who forgives all your iniquities, Who heals all your diseases, Who redeems your life from destruction, Who crowns you with lovingkindness and tender mercies, Who satisfies your mouth with good things, So that your youth is renewed like the eagle's (Psalm 103:1–5 NKJV).

Jun & Joy Yuko, Japan

Tuesday, March 4 — Fighting Three Kinds of Battle

A friend recently told me I would have to fight this battle on three different levels, and I am beginning to experience the reality of that statement.

She said I would have to fight on a spiritual level. This is probably the easiest for me, as it is the one of which I am most familiar. I find confidence with much gratitude in the knowledge that many of you are fighting the spiritual battle *with* me, and sometimes *for* me.

I am confident in God's love, His constant presence, and His power to heal. I gain strength and comfort from His Word, daily. He gives me encouragement and guidance. I know how to stand against the enemy, and am grateful for the weapons the Lord has given to me to fight the spiritual battle and for the armor that protects me.

I am also fighting this battle on an emotional level, but I don't remember ever having any training in this area. I am asking the Lord to show me how.

When I visited the oncologist a couple of weeks ago and was told chemotherapy was the recommended treatment, the oncologist said that hair loss is one of the side effects. I knew that and had already fought that battle on the spiritual level. One Wednesday evening during worship at church, we sang an old hymn I had not heard in years, *I Surrender All.*[3] As I sang, I knew the Lord was looking at my heart to see if I meant what I was singing. Before the song was over, He reminded me, "You are not your hair." My hair does not have eternal value. I had to take another step of surrender — of both my hair and my vanity! The result was His precious, priceless inner peace that flooded my soul.

Even when I deal with things in the spiritual realm, I still have to walk through emotional situations. I know my emotions in themselves are not good or bad, but I don't want them to control my life, my actions, my decisions, or my choices. I want the Spirit of God to be in control.

For example, last Friday I experienced an emotional battle. Carie and Christie took me to order a wig. My emotions were rebelling. I didn't want to go, and my emotions fought against my making a decision. I tried on several wigs but was not impressed. In fact, I was discouraged, was praying like crazy for patience, and was about to decide that a "do-rag" was the best option after all. Then, the young lady put another wig on me, and I cried. I knew it was the right wig . . . even though it was blonde. (No, I am actually NOT going to be blonde, though it was tempting! I ordered the wig in my own hair color.)

By the time we left the store, I knew I had persevered. I was grateful, encouraged, exhausted, glad it was done, and hungry. Carie and Christie took me to lunch and we talked and laughed. Truly, *"A joyful heart is good medicine . . ."* (Proverbs 17:22 NASB).

The third level of battle is in the physical realm. Someday in the future, my hair will fall out. I cannot control that, but I will walk through it, hopefully with grace and maybe even with a sense of humor. I am fighting the physical battle by doing what is necessary each day. (Today, I had my hair cut very short in preparation for what is ahead.) Most of all, I am doing what the doctors tell me to do, knowing that they want me to be healed and they have the expertise to get me through this physically.

My friend says that I will win on all levels of battle. But even when the children of Israel entered the land that the Lord had promised to them, they had to possess the land by fighting the giants (Deuteronomy 1:21, 28-30). I am walking in God's promises knowing that victory is assured, but I am also fighting the giants. Thank you for your prayers and support and for fighting the giants with me. I could not do this without you.

❧ GUEST

How precious to read your thoughts as you bare your soul through an open book—so valuable. It sows seed of honesty, openness, and humility. It prepares readers for similar experiences—God never meant for us to walk alone. But when we keep personal, important things to ourselves, no one benefits, including the one with the secrets who gives no opportunity for encouragement or wisdom from would-be supporters.

So thank you for being vulnerable to us—sharing your hurdles, the victories, humor, and perseverance. You share tools we can build with!

I appreciate Carie and Christie and their support. I am sure God smiles, seeing the three of you together.

Love and hugs to you all, with prayers,

Dianna

❧ GUEST

"The Lord does not look at the things man looks at. Man looks at the outward appearance, but the Lord looks at the heart" (1 Samuel 16:7b). God must surely be pleased with your heart.

Love you,
Sarah

❧ GUEST

Once again, as I read your journal entry, I recognized that God is coordinating the prayers being offered on your behalf.

I also recalled how you have always said you did not want to settle for what was good; you wanted only God's best for you. I believe that all through this journey, you will receive only God's best for you — from the top of your head to the soles of your feet. And that includes your hair!

I love you!
Linda

Thursday, March 6—Unexpected Surgery

During my first surgery, the surgeon removed several lymph nodes which contained cancer cells. Tomorrow at noon, I will have a second surgery. The surgeon will remove more nodes under my right arm. There are three levels of lymph nodes and the surgeon will remove two levels — a possible 20-30 nodes. She will also insert a "port" on the left side of my chest. The port has a wire that goes into a heart vein. I will receive chemotherapy through the port.

I was originally told that if it was necessary to remove the additional lymph nodes, that would be done during the first surgery. After I came out of recovery in February, Charlie told me that I might have to undergo another surgery. The surgeon said that the pathologist was not able to complete all of the necessary tests during my surgery, so they would have to wait for his final report before they would know if further surgery would be required. For the first time during this journey, I was discouraged. I was not prepared for a second surgery.

Charlie and Christie left the room to get coffee, and Carie was with me. I needed for her to pray for me. Her prayer reminded me of what I know: God, not the doctors, is in control of my life. He has a plan and it is a good plan with a future and a hope (Jeremiah 29:11). He does all things with purpose and out of His great love and care.

Hindsight is an amazing thing. I once told Charlie that hindsight is such a special gift that I was certain it had to be in the Bible, and I was going to find it. And I did. Many times, the Lord told His disciples things that He knew they would not understand until much later (John 12:16; 13:7, 19; 14:29; 16:4). Hindsight is when we look back and finally understand.

As I reflect on the past three weeks since the first surgery, I now see what a gift the extra time has been. I have been able to move forward in recovering from the first surgery and am stronger to face the second one. I have taken steps that are necessary to prepare for the future: I ordered "Wanda the wig," cut my hair, met the wonderful people in the oncologist's office, toured the treatment room, went through tests necessary before chemotherapy begins, and set the date for the first and second treatments. The oncologist worked with me to arrange my treatments around my schedule so that I can travel to New Mexico in April to speak at a women's retreat! I have had time to do some things around the house. (Today, I am defrosting the freezer—haven't done this kind of "nesting" since I was about to have a baby—decades ago!) I have spent precious time with my grandchildren who have needed fun, face-to-face time with Grammy. And I had three additional weeks to pray about tomorrow's surgery.

It would have been easy for me to stay discouraged and upset with the situation. Often our tendency is to go into a "victim mentality" when things do not go as we would have planned. But I thank the Lord for His truth and wisdom that sets us free and brings hope. He truly has a perfect plan and a perfect timing. He can be trusted.

The surgeon apologized that I must undergo surgery again, but she was not willing to remove the lymph nodes unless she was certain that it was necessary. I told her that many people were praying that she would have wisdom and that we know God answers prayer. I believe she made the best decision. By tomorrow morning, I will be ready for the next step of the healing process.

Before Christmas, Charlie and I went to several parties where we exchanged "white elephant gifts." Almost every time, my gift included packages of Kleenex®. A friend sent me a Christmas gift, and in the package were beautiful decorative tissues. I asked the Lord why I was getting all these tissues, but I didn't get an answer. A couple of weeks ago, a friend sent me some special gifts from a Moravian settlement on the east coast and included in the package were more tissues. I finally understood. The tissues are next to my computer. As I read the encouraging things you write to me, I am using the tissues to wipe my tears. Your words touch my heart. May the Lord somehow impress on you what I cannot adequately express, how much your words bring life and joy!

❧ GUEST

Good morning, Sis!

I guess I'll be the first to write today. Glad you found a wig that you like. I have my Dolly Parton wig right here ready to bring when I come to visit. We will both put on our wigs and laugh at each other. Of course, yours will look correct, but you can just imagine an old fat man with a Dolly Parton wig. . . .

I know you are prepared for the next few days. I have been focusing on this all week as you asked. Our friend had no nerve damage with her surgery, so I expect yours to go even better than hers did. After all, she just had a little country doctor doing her work.

I'll not try to quote Scriptures as you know them better than I do. I'll just say that we are praying for you as you move toward your day with the doc. Don't forget your socks!

Love,
JB

Friday, March 7 — Surgery Recovery

Dad, Christie, and I (Carie) are with Mom in her recovery room. We wanted to send out an update. Mom's surgeon said the surgery went well. Mom's port is in place, and the surgeon removed the lymph nodes. We don't know how many, but the amount of tissue was minimal. The surgeon reported that she did not encounter any major nerves during the surgery. Also, she installed the port with no complications.

The surgeon believes that Mom's healing will go quickly and without much pain. Thank you for your prayers and especially those targeting the potential complications of today's surgery. God is answering.

Mom is resting now. She is experiencing some pain, so we ask that you continue to pray for relief. Otherwise, she looks great, and we are thanking God for His presence in the hospital today and His faithful healing hand that Mom rested in during surgery.

The anesthesiologist called last night to discuss today's procedure. As he and Mom were talking, she told him that many people were praying for him and for all those who would be in the operating room. His reply was that if she believed that God was in control during the surgery, she would do well. He was right!

Sunday, March 9 — Recovering and Preparing for the Next Step

It is Sunday morning, and a beautiful day outside — mid 50s, sun shining, and blue sky — especially nice after an unusual week with two snows. Charlie left for church a few minutes ago. I am sitting at my desk looking out over the pastures. The water tank in the back pasture is full of water again, our garden is growing, the grass is turning green, wildflowers are beginning to bloom, and the birds are outside singing. All of this is wonderful as it makes me feel very much alive.

I appreciate that Carie sent you an update from the hospital. As she already told you, surgery went well. THANK YOU for your specific prayers! So far, I have no numbness in my arm or hand. That is answer to my prayer.

I came home from the hospital Friday evening, about six hours after surgery. I had almost no pain and slept soundly all night, except to turn off the alarm and take medication. Yesterday, I got up feeling like I could live a normal day. Then I quickly remembered that I was on pain medication and it was doing its job! I decided that I had better be wise and rest, so I actually slept part of the day. (A friend prayed that I would have a "napping anointing"! Napping is not something I often do.)

Charlie had a meeting yesterday, so Carie and our granddaughter Rebekah came over to take care of me. Rebekah allowed me to beat her at a card game, and we watched a movie. Carie studied, fixed lunch, and cleaned my kitchen. Chris, Christie, and Cella came over yesterday evening to bring a yummy dinner that friends provided.

The next step, chemotherapy, doesn't start for almost a month. I am grateful for time to recover from the surgeries and to prepare my mind and heart. Chemotherapy is a *big unknown* to me, but I am grateful that the One who controls my life is *much bigger*. The Lord reminded me of an obvious fact that I needed to hear: nothing that will happen in my body will impact, influence, or change Him. He will be the same inside of me as He has always been. His power will not decrease. His love will be as strong. He will be with me (Romans 8:38–39). He will never leave me. He knows everything and is able to control and direct all that happens in me. His words bring comfort for this season of preparation.

I am very grateful to be this far along in the healing process.

I am overwhelmed by all the love I have received. I have never liked the greeting cards that say, "Although I never say it . . .." I always want to respond with, "Just say it!" And you have. Your words build me up, bless me, and bring me strength and joy. "Thank you" seems so small and does not express my gratitude. I pray that the Lord reward you greatly for all you have done to encourage me.

❧ GUEST

I am reminded of how you and Charlie prayed and stood by me during my bout with cancer last year. Your steadfast faith, strength, and love encouraged me to fight and focus on the truth of Jesus. I pray for your continued strength and know that the Lord has you in His arms. Know that Constance and I love you very much and pray believing for your complete healing.

Shalom!
Woodrow

❧ GUEST

I love your latest message, Mom. As you go through this struggle, you continue to amaze me as you keep your eyes on the Creator and remember His goodness, faithfulness, consistency. I learn so much from you and thank you for the spiritual legacy that you and

Daddy have placed before me and have claimed for my children and (someday) grandchildren. What a jewel for the kingdom you are, and how much I appreciate all of these friends who recognize your value and hold you dear in prayer. Sleep well, darling mother and friend! I'll see you tomorrow.

Carie

Tuesday, March 11 — Praying for Patience

I had a follow-up appointment with the surgeon this morning and all is going well in healing from both surgeries. I have decreased the amount of pain medication that I am taking, and my system is beginning to stabilize. I will not see the surgeon again for six months.

I experienced a miracle today. I have been praying that the drain would come out by next Friday, which would be one week after surgery. After my first surgery, I had the drain for 10 days, which seemed very l-o-n-g. But, today—on the fourth day—the surgeon removed the drain. I am rejoicing! Now I can shower again! YEAH! So basic, yet such a luxury.

The surgeon said that during the second surgery, she removed only six lymph nodes, which is pretty amazing. All six were cancer free. I have not experienced any lymphedema (swelling in my arm), and she does not expect any. She said for me to begin to exercise. These are specific answers to your prayers.

Chemotherapy treatment begins in four weeks. I am not ready and, thankfully, don't have to be ready today. God's timing in all these things is perfect, and He is preparing me for one step at a time.

In December, before the cancer was discovered, I knew that my primary prayer for the next year would be for patience. Part of learning patience is to walk in God's timing and not get ahead of Him. Each day, I am seeking His plan for that day. I think that is called the patient's patience!

Yesterday's plan was for me to spend the day resting, which is something I don't do easily. I am learning to stop pushing myself, to take care of my body and to conserve my energy. It is a matter of self-discipline, another area in which I must grow.

Thank you again for your prayers. I hope you understand the power of your prayers and, even more so, the power of God, as His hand moves when you pray.

A friend gave me Dutch Sheets' book *Authority in Prayer*[4], and it is truly one of those "for-such-a-time-as-this" books for me. I have walked through the past two and a half months wrapped in God's peace and His loving presence. Cancer has not controlled my life, and I have not bowed to the fears, doubts, and questions that could have controlled my thinking and diverted my attention. Truly, God is being sovereign over my life, my thoughts, and my expectations during this time.

Yet, from here, it looks like the road is about to become steeper, and I am going to be stretched in the coming months. The Lord is already bringing the necessary preparation and equipping into my life for what is ahead.

Thank you for the valuable and precious gift that each of you is to me and to my family in this season of my life. May the Lord richly reward you for your love, encouragement, and your service to Him and to His children.

❧ GUEST

How good our Father is! Those things that He is developing in you, He is developing in me. Testimonies of His faithfulness are always encouraging. My story is different but our direction the same. How precious and gentle is our Shepherd who leads us beside still waters in green pastures. We have no other friend like Him who walks with us all the way and has already suffered for us. How humbling is God's goodness.

> Love and hugs,
> Dianna

❧ GUEST

Praise God for such wonderful healing! It sounds like you're doing great. Drain out in four days? I'm jealous! :)

I know that chemo looks like a huge mountain in front of you, but you will be on the other side of it before you know it. I made it through eight rounds and I know you can do it, too. Just take it one day at a time—sometimes one *hour* at a time.

I will pray that your patience continues to grow and that God will continue to reveal Himself to you every day.

> Susan

I thank God that you are not allowing cancer to be lord of your life. That is a powerful statement. We praise Him for the faithfulness He continues to show to you and to us through you at this time. Thank you for all you are allowing Him to do in and through you and especially for the testimony of your daily walk with Him. Glory to God in the Highest.

Love,
Darleen

Thursday, March 13 — Caregivers

Many of you have said you are especially praying for Charlie, Carie, and Christie — the "care-givers." Thank you. I watch them, and especially Charlie, give sacrificially on a daily basis, as he continues with all of his normal responsibilities and then does much more. Charlie and the girls have gone to doctor appointments, asked questions, studied information about breast cancer and options for treatment on the Internet, taken time to listen to me express my feelings and needs, fixed and delivered meals, and done many practical things. Charlie helps with the cooking, washing dishes, cleaning, and doing laundry and even helps me get dressed at times. The other day, he offered to help me shampoo before I went to the doctor.

Many times in the past few months, Charlie has stopped what he was doing to simply sit down and listen to me. Sometimes, he comes into my office and knows that I am struggling with something. He sits on the windowsill and takes this position, with his arms folded and a look of patience on his face that says, "I am here to listen if you need me." He listens without having to "fix me" or the situation. If needed, he gives encouragement or a word of wisdom. And he has a sensitive understanding of when I need to be alone to think things through. He allows me to do what I have strength to do, knowing that I need to feel useful. Then he picks up the slack and does what I cannot do.

I am not going through this journey alone. I spend much time praying for those who do walk alone. This journey is affecting my entire family. My desire is to be an encouragement to them, and that they, too, will be closer to Jesus when this is over. I am asking the Lord to build their faith through this time of testing, as He is building mine.

Charlie and I have precious friends who have been on my heart much in the past couple of weeks. In many ways, they have been like parents to us for the past 25 years. We met when they attended a Bible class that Charlie was teaching at our home church. Several years ago, the wife went into the hospital. After treatment, the doctor would not release her to go home, only to assisted living. In a matter of a few weeks, her husband sold the beautiful home he had designed and built for her, sold their belongings, and moved into a two-room assisted-living apartment. He could still drive but was required to give up his vehicle so that he could live in the facility with his wife.

We visit them when we go to their city. We pick up dinner at Luby's and spend the evening eating, fellowshipping, reminiscing, laughing, and sharing the good things that God is doing in our lives. Often, Charlie serves them communion and we have a time of prayer. This couple has spent many years praying for us and encouraging our ministry.

The husband's focus has been to care for and encourage his wife. He is an amazing example of a loving caregiver and friend. He is always joyful, positive, and compassionate, and we have never heard him complain. He always has words of praise and encouragement.

This morning, we received a call that the wife has gone to be with the Lord. We rejoice that she is with Jesus, but we pray for her husband and children. He must now work to build a life without her and that will be difficult after being married for 60 years.

So, I thank you for praying for Charlie and the girls as they care for me. They are a special gift of God to my life. Please continue to pray for their encouragement, health, and strength and for God's grace to be upon them.

❧ GUEST

Thank you for sharing from the family perspective. I commend Charlie as he accompanies you on this journey. Listening is a gift, a ministry.

Your journal entry of how your whole family is affected by your condition reminded me that we are all one body, connected and never meant to function in isolation. Surely, God longs for us to see ourselves that way: to honor others as better than ourselves and to pray when another suffers. Being members of Christ's body makes us members belonging to all the other body parts — "So in

Christ we who are many form one body, and each member belongs to all the others" (Romans 12:5). That statement holds much meaning. May Christ be honored as we relate to one another.

With love and hugs,
Dianna

❧ GUEST

I love reading your journal entries. Thanks for taking your intimate feelings and sharing them with us. Cella and I had a good discussion at the mall last night (in between "Oh, Mom, can we buy this?" and "Oh, Mama, can we get a snack?" Ha!) about why God allows things to happen, even if those things make us sad. Cella's answer to the question in regard to you was simply, "Well, Grammy is getting to see how much we love her more than ever, so maybe God just thought she needed a little more love right now." I don't know how theologically sound her answer is (smile), but you are definitely seeing an outpouring of love that has been there all along but just hasn't been shown so deliberately before. Mom, may we all be so blessed to be loved like you are loved. And may we all be so willing to love others the way you do.

Christie

Monday, March 17 — Responding Culturally to Breast Cancer

I used to think that I had personal experience with cancer. My grandmother died of cancer. My aunt had cancer. My mother was diagnosed with cancer when I was 19 years old. She died less than a year later, only weeks after Charlie and I were married. However, recently, my definition of "personal experience" has changed.

In the past two and a half months, I have begun a "crash course" in a subject I rarely noticed before. The doctors have given me stacks of books and pamphlets to read. Initially, I was easily overwhelmed with more information than I wanted or needed. I am learning to take one step at a time, and to read only the information that I need for the next step.

When you have cancer, as with many crises in life, you suddenly have much information to assimilate, many decisions to make, numerous issues to deal with, and lots of questions to answer. It is personal and life changing. I will never be the same again. I am being forced to make changes that will affect the rest of my life. That is not necessarily a bad thing but can be overwhelming and emotional when confronted with all of this unexpectedly and in a short time.

As I am trying to make decisions and assimilate information, I find it difficult to answer questions that many people have about my situation. Cancer has become a personal issue. It has become an emotional issue. I find I am having a hard time with what sometimes feels like a "casual or curious approach" to the subject.

Christie helped me understand when she reminded me that breast cancer has become a very open issue in the United States. Is has become too common in women and has received much media attention. The result includes many positive things, especially increased communication, preventive health care, awareness, and education. However, as an issue becomes more public and is talked about so openly, often privacy and sensitivity decreases or disappears.

Recently, I have seen another, and almost opposite, approach to breast cancer that greatly disturbs me. Christie was at a meeting where the speaker was talking specifically about perspectives of breast cancer in other nations. She shared that in many Middle East nations, when a woman is diagnosed with breast cancer, society rejects her. Her husband often abandons her and remarries, and, because of the possibility of the cancer being hereditary, her daughters will never marry.

I have often taken for granted my wedding vows that included "for better or for worse, in sickness and in health." Those vows have become even more precious as I have seen Charlie walk through this situation with me. He says that whatever affects me affects him. That committed support is a priceless gift that many women in the world do not have.

Among the books that the oncologist gave me, one had a long chapter that focused specifically on how to handle being diagnosed with cancer and having your husband leave because he could not handle the situation. I realized that this must be common, even in America, or it would not have been included in the book, but the fact that it was necessary grieved me. I cannot imagine being abandoned when you need the support the most, but I now realize this does happen.

An article in the *Dallas Morning News*[5] recently addressed women with breast cancer in other nations. A local Methodist minister, a survivor of breast cancer herself, met with a delegation to the U.S. who were guests of the U.S. State Department. The delegates were either survivors of breast cancer, physicians, or nurses from countries such as Syria, Libya, Egypt, and Bahrain. In their own nations, many of the women do not have the freedom to talk about this disease. They said that many women with breast cancer will choose to die quietly, denying or ignoring the disease because of the social stigma associated with it and because their cultures say they got the disease because they did something wrong. One doctor said that these countries don't have advocacy, media, or breast-care centers and have a shortage of medicine. In Asia and other parts of the world, many people remain silent on the issue. Patients have little or no support.

I was ignorant about this issue until recently. As for the facts that I need to know to make intelligent decisions about my health and my future, I may forget those after my need for the information is gone. After I have completed the recommended cancer treatment, I will adjust to any permanent changes that having cancer brings to my life. But as for these women around the world and the many ways their lives are affected, I will not easily forget them.

When I think of all that is available to us in America — technology, medication, information, educated doctors, caring nurses, even laws that require insurance companies to pay for wigs and other necessities — I find it difficult to complain. I am not trivializing difficult situations. Many of you have walked through more challenging situations than I am facing, and you have walked in faith and grace. Your lives have been an encouragement to me. We each have to walk through difficult places in life.

Even though chemotherapy presently seems like a huge mountain ahead of me, as I think of the people suffering and dying because treatment is not available, I thank the Lord for all that is being done to bring about my healing. And when I weep, it is most often for those who are alone and who live in fear and silence because of their culture's perspective of this disease. I will spend much of the rest of my life praying for those women who have little or no hope.

These issues weigh heavily on my heart. Thanks to you who are walking with me through this season of life. I cannot tell you how grateful I am that we, as Americans, are not silenced and living in fear like so many people around the world. And again, thank you for the support and love you give me that so many people do not have. Your messages continue to encourage me. You are a treasured gift and you will never know what a big difference you are making in my life.

✣ *GUEST*

My prayers are with you and your family. I can only imagine what a change this is for you. God has shown me this past year that change is inevitable but that He never changes and He always keeps His promises. Jeremiah 29:11–13 is a real comfort to me and I wanted to share that with you. You and Charlie continue to bless and inspire, and God will be glorified through this trial. Thank you for being willing to share your journey.

Love to you and your family,

Debbie

✣ *GUEST*

I know that when God takes you through something, He will sustain and uphold you in that place. Praise God that He is taking you *through*. He never leaves us nor forsakes us. Be blessed and walk in the favor of the Lord.

Darlene

✣ *GUEST*

Thank you so much for sharing the course that you are traveling. We need to hear those things so that we may better know Christ, the power of His resurrection, and the fellowship of His sufferings (Philippians 3:10).

God creatively brings me in contact with people for the purpose of prayer. I have seen that as a pattern. I have learned to pray for my children's' friends, neighbors, business associates, and even for other drivers who come into my path on the road. When I am ready to blast my horn, I remember that there is a higher purpose.

So we are each drawn into another realm where prayer needs are laid out for us. I was unaware of the plight of women in other nations who suffer like this. Now I'm in a church with its own set of prayer needs!

Your friendship, your ministry (it's just part of your life, whatever you are doing) are gifts that I treasure. May our Father bring discernment and grace as you plow through all the information and options before you so that your decisions are a result of God's wisdom.

Love and hugs,
Dianna

❧ GUEST

Our little church has people from various backgrounds. Several mentioned that they wanted to know more about fasting. So in preparation for teaching a class on the subject, I read all the Scripture passages regarding fasting and tried to remember what you had taught me. I was greatly helped by Beth Alves' teaching in *The Mighty Warrior*[6] and Arthur Wallis' *God's Chosen Fast*[7]. I was particularly struck by Wallis' statement regarding Elijah's fast during his preparation for ministry. Elijah ate bread and meat brought to him by ravens and he drank water from a brook. Then he went to the home of the widow of Zarephath where he ate cakes made with meal and oil. Elijah's fast was simple and lean because there was a famine in the land. Wallis said, "To minister effectively to those in need, we must be identified with their need and sit where they sit … God never fails to honor such self-denial" (p. 23).

When I read your journal entry yesterday, I was struck by the knowledge that you are being given concerning the "famine" that the women of the world are experiencing in regard to their battle with breast cancer. I was touched with the fact that you are now "sitting where they sit." I wonder if God is preparing you to minister to these women?

I love you and your family for the blessings I have received through your obedience to the leading of the Holy Spirit. May you delight in the Lord and experience His presence today in a new and beautiful way.

Linda

Saturday, March 22 — Looking Beyond the Present Situation

My heart is very grateful for the timing of what I am going through. God has used Christmas, New Year's, the end of winter, the coming of spring, and now Easter to speak to me about my present life journey.

There is an element of God that is *externally visible* in nature, if we will only stop and take notice. I see evidence of His presence daily as I sit in my office looking at the pastures and tree lines that are being transformed one step at a time, as they go from barrenness of winter that looks like death to being full of life, color, and fruit.

Even more, His presence *within me* is evident as He is sustaining me. His words of guidance, assurance, love, and wisdom are guarding me from those things that seek to kill my hope, confidence, courage, and faith.

I have shared with you that from the beginning of this situation, I did not fear cancer. That is amazing. And I do not fear death. I am spending my life preparing for the eternal life that is ahead. So what the world calls "death" is actually "promotion day" for me as a Christian.

However, recently I have found that chemotherapy seems insurmountable. For several weeks, I have not been able to see beyond it. This surprised me since cancer comes to kill, but the treatment is intended to heal and protect me from further disease. Yet chemotherapy, for me, has been the more difficult and fearful challenge to face.

In the past week, I have even come close to refusing treatment, though I know in my heart what I am to do. Some of you have asked about specifics and dates of that treatment and I have not been able to respond because I am not yet ready for that part of the journey.

This week I have been reading about the treatment, the drugs, and potential side effects. The enormity of it has been overwhelming. A young woman—a doctor's wife, mother of young children, and a friend of Carie's—is helping me. She has been through many more surgeries and treatment than I will undergo. Her doctors are the same doctors who are treating me, and her testimony of their ability and sensitivity has been an added blessing. She is encouraging me by sharing her experience, emotions, questions, preparation, facts about cancer and treatment, ways to prevent some of the side effects, and, above all, God's faithfulness to her through the process.

In the past two days, I have begun to have breakthrough concerning treatment. As I have meditated on the Scriptures and listened to the Lord's encouragement, I am gaining a vision of "beyond treatment" — not only in time but also in magnitude. I have finally seen the Lord as being much larger than what I am going through. That probably should be obvious to me. But my understanding of familiar truths is growing even deeper. For this new challenge, I need new understanding of God and His character.

In my mind, I know God is bigger than my situation. But until *knowledge sinks into my heart* and becomes personal and real for the present situation, it does little good. In fact, sometimes when I know things only in my head, I experience confusion, turmoil, and discontent. I have to "press in" in order to *live* in the full experience of God that is available to me as a Christian. The pressing in is different for each circumstance, because the Lord rarely does things the same way twice. His methods change. Yet, His character is consistent and He answers as I pray and then wait, listening for His voice.

This week, through focusing on the death and resurrection of Christ, I have seen the familiar truths of Easter take a fresh new relevance in my life. His death on the cross was a complete work. His work and my salvation are intended to have practical and relevant impact on the daily issues of my life. He has provided all I need.

The reality of His sacrifice in Isaiah 53:5 (NKJV) is very personal: "He *was* wounded for [*my*] transgressions, He *was* bruised for [*my*] iniquities; the chastisement for [*my*] peace (well-being) *was* upon Him, and *by His stripes [I] am healed*" (emphasis added). This is all *past* provision accomplished 2,000 years ago on the cross but is available for me to claim by faith for my life today, throughout treatment, and every day after.

Another personally challenging Scripture speaks of Jesus: ". . . who for the joy set before Him endured the cross . . ." (Hebrews 12:2 NASB). Jesus had a vision of something beyond the beatings, scourging, and even the crucifixion that gave Him the ability to walk through the horrible reality of the moment.

Jesus did not avoid the cross, but He went through it. Even more difficult than death on the cross was separation from His Father ("My God, my God, why have you forsaken me?" [Mark 15:34b].) He experienced that separation so I would not. He experienced "spiritual death" for me. I pray that I will walk in the reality of His sacrifice in a way that will bring joy to Him.

With His example before me, I am amazed at how joy has started to help me look beyond the treatment. The joy is taking me beyond the fear of the unknown, perhaps because I am once again focusing on truth that *is known*—the ever-present care, steadfast promises, power, all-mightiness, and love of God.

Thank you for indulging me in my "thinking out loud" and speaking from my heart. Journaling is helping me to be honest about where I am and to get where I need to be. I am experiencing many new emotions, questions, weaknesses, insights, and understandings. This is a journey like nothing I have ever walked through before.

Perhaps what I have shared will help you to know how to pray for me. My focus is on the present — on what I have to do today. I still have several weeks before I begin treatment, and I want to be mentally, emotionally, physically, and spiritually prepared.

May the reality of the cross and the resurrection be fresh, personal, and relevant to you this weekend and in the days following. As Charlie and I are celebrating the personal reality of Easter, may you also celebrate with deeper experience and revelation of His love and provision for your lives.

❧ GUEST

I have been reading your journals and remembering how fervently you would take notes at church. Today, Easter Sunday, I went to church with friends and began writing down some of the pastor's comments — about what Jesus did on the cross for us. Jesus himself was perfect, yet took *all* our sins and sickness upon Himself. I do not think my mind fully fathoms the greatness of what He did.

I remember one time at church, we were singing . . . "I Could Sing of Your Love Forever"[8] and I understood that we can sing that song because *His love lasts forever*. Such is the love Jesus has for *you*. I was also aware that we needed to sing with all our might because we were singing to God Almighty. I felt so inadequate in expressing what it really meant to sing to an *Almighty God*.

I will continue [to] pray for you!

Michelle

Monday, March 24 — Overcoming Fear and Wearing My New Wig

Last week was spring break for our grandchildren, and Charlie and I spent some quality time with them. They came out to "the farm" and had a wonderful time playing in the mud, pretending to be pirates, sword fighting with sticks, gathering old tree branches, and helping PawPaw put branches in the "chipper-shredder" to make mulch for the garden. They played Yahtzee™ with Grammy, dyed eggs, watched movies, and ate and talked a lot! It was fun.

One of my desires is that, as our grandchildren see me walk through this healing process, they will grow in faith and not in fear. Charlie taught at church last Wednesday evening and made the statement, *"There is no fear in faith, and there is no faith in fear."* When I am afraid, I am putting my faith in the plan of the enemy rather than in God and His plan.

I want my life to demonstrate to my children and grandchildren the reality that God is faithful and completely trustworthy. So I have determined to deal with every fear that arises. As I see God's hand move on my behalf, it builds my faith and increases thanksgiving and praise in my heart. And as His love removes the fear in my heart, it demonstrates His amazing power. That is the inheritance I want to leave for my family.

I have one friend in particular who, when she heard that I was diagnosed with breast cancer, responded with tremendous fear. When I asked her why, she recalled that as a small child, she watched her mother's closest friend go through sickness and death from breast cancer. That experience impacted her life in such a way that, as an adult, she is still reacting in fear.

Her story encouraged me to pray that our children and grandchildren would have a different experience and testimony. I want my family to see the truth—that the power of God is greater than the power of the enemy. We do not need to be afraid. Instead, we can trust God. For me to pray this with faith and without fear, I must live it in the situations of my own life.

It seems that some of our fears are a result of the "unknown," so I am trying to be open with our children and grandchildren. They are the only ones to whom I have said that they can ask me any question and I will answer it.

When Carie told her children that I was going to lose my hair, Nathaniel asked, "Is Grammy going to be a 'baldy'?" Carie told him "Yes," but added that it might hurt a lady's feelings to be called that. Nathaniel answered, "Okay!" That was the end of that conversation. However, the girls were especially concerned. So last week, Carie and I decided to include them in the trip to pick up my new wig. We thought that would be great fun for them.

The "wig man" cut and styled my "new hair" and informed me that the name of my wig is "Peaches" (not "Wanda the Wig"). So I will be wearing Peaches for months to come. When I arrived home wearing my new wig, Charlie just thought I had a new hairdo.

I decided to wear my new wig to church on Easter Sunday. It was amazing how many people, instead of immediately asking how I was feeling, said how good I looked and how much they liked my new hair cut! Several said they liked my new style better than the old one! I simply said, "Thank you!" It was very refreshing for my health to not be the subject of conversation.

God looks at the heart, not the outward appearance of man (I Samuel 16:7). But more often people see only the outside. I am encouraged that I can go through the next few months and (I hope) people will not see a "sick lady." At church, as we sang "It Is Well with My Soul"[9], I could sing and mean it. Inside, God is ministering to and building my soul and spirit.

In the physical, I don't feel sick. The cancerous tumor is gone and I am recovering from surgery. Each day, I feel better and I am gaining strength. And I have taken some giant steps in dealing with my attitude toward the coming treatment.

Truly, Christ is risen, and the power of His death, His life and His resurrection is as effective today as it was that first Easter. I celebrate and rejoice with you over all the amazing things God has done for us. And my heart overflows with gratitude for relationship—relationship with Him and with you.

GUEST

Cella loved her time with you and PawPaw on Easter and thinks you're the "best-est ever Grammy in the world!" She asked if Chris could have some of your medicine that makes hair fall out because he has a lot of hair in his nose that he needs to get rid of! HA! You looked stunning on Sunday and had an air of confidence and strength about you. We loved sharing the time with you.

Pardon for sin and a peace that endureth,
Thy own dear presence to cheer and to guide;
Strength for today and bright hope for tomorrow,
Blessings all mine, with ten thousand beside!

"Great is Thy faithfulness!" "Great is Thy faithfulness!"
Morning by morning new mercies I see;
All I have needed Thy hand hath provided—
"Great is Thy faithfulness," Lord, unto me![10]

Christie

You're right that what's on the inside is the most important part of who we are, but I also believe that doing things to maintain your outward appearance during treatments will make a big difference in how you feel about yourself. I vowed early on that I would never look like a cancer patient. Any time I left the house, I wore my wig, applied my makeup, wore a cute outfit (when physically possible), and put on some of my favorite jewelry—even to my chemo treatments.

Everyone has her own way of dealing with the changes in appearance that chemo brings, but it was my way of taking control of something. It really made me feel good when I looked in the mirror; I saw a healthy-looking person.

God will be right by your side all the way through chemo. You can do it together!

Susan

Tuesday, March 25 — Climbing the Mountain

(Precious friends . . . Thank you again for your love and encouragement—those treasured words of life! The tissues remain next to my computer! [sniff] Please know that your words don't just make me cry; they also bring strength.)

Yesterday, a friend sent me powerful words she had researched about mountains. I am digesting them. Then this morning—I am confident that it was not by coincidence but God's divine direction—a friend sent the following poem. God has given her a unique gift of words that has touched my heart many times in the past 12 years, and her poems always come at the right time. May this be a blessing to you as you "climb" your mountain.

> My Destiny Is JESUS
>
> I have climbed the rocky mountain
> I have scaled its steepest wall;
> Even when it wasn't easy
> And I thought I'd surely fall.

But, no matter how discouraged,
Continued in the climb;
It's like my faith propelled me higher
Than the doubts that plagued my mind.

I believe that unseen angels
Were dispersed to carry me;
As I struggled up the mountain
Toward my promised destiny.

You see, my journey takes me upward
To the foot of heaven's throne;
And so, I cannot lose my vision
Nor allow my thoughts to roam.

Today, I'm just a pilgrim
Traveling through a foreign land;
But My Destiny is JESUS
And He will always hold my hand.

So, I'll continue this life's journey
And climb the mountain wall;
I will keep my focus, steady
Knowing, HE, won't let me fall!

—Terese Holloway[11]

Thank you, Terese, for this powerful and confirming word. Keep listening to the Lord and may those words continue to touch many other lives as they have touched mine!

Friday, March 28 — Facing the Upcoming Schedule

My first praise is that my recovery from surgery continues to progress. I am exercising and have regained much of the motion in my arm, and my physical strength improves daily.

Also, this week I have had some breakthrough in my heart toward the upcoming treatment. In taking one step at a time, facing chemotherapy came to the top of the list; I knew it was time to deal with it. The fact that I can openly write about it shows that I have made progress. This week, I have read about (and prayed over) the details of the treatment and potential side effects. I have also researched what I can do to help limit the side effects. I am not yet ready but have taken a big step forward. I am grateful for how the Lord is preparing me. Please continue to pray that I will be ready.

Here is what is presently on my schedule in the next 10 days:

After the doctor received the results of a heart scan that I had several weeks ago, he scheduled me for a heart sonogram next Monday.

On Wednesday, April 2, I have a preparatory appointment with the oncologist.

On Tuesday morning, April 8, I will begin chemotherapy. I plan to be in the clinic for five hours.

The second treatment is scheduled for April 29. The weekend before, I will speak at a women's retreat in New Mexico. Carie is going with me, and I am trusting the Lord to give me the energy and strength for that ministry. I am excited and looking forward to it.

I do not yet have dates for following treatments. As I understand the process, I will visit the oncologist's office regularly between treatments because he will monitor things like my blood count. If all goes the way the oncologist (and the patient!) prefers, treatments will be every three weeks, and I will be finished with chemotherapy by the end of the summer.

In the meantime, I have a long list of projects I am trying to complete before treatment begins. I will be unable to do a number of things once I begin chemotherapy, so I am working now to accomplish as much my energy allows.

Thank you for your prayers. I believe God is answering them in abundance. I continue to feel God's presence and walk in His amazing peace. I am grateful for your love, support, and encouragement. Your friendship makes a big difference.

GUEST

> . . . and your friendship makes a difference in our lives. . . . Someone once mentioned how many lives are touched when any one person comes into the world. . . . I was quite surprised because the number was about 10,000 people affected by one life. . . . Your life is touching many more.

With love,
Darleen

I will be eager to hear how God showed His faithfulness at your doctor's appointment today. I thought of you when I read the verse that says, "He will never leave you nor forsake you" (Deuteronomy 31:6b).

Do you know what "forsake" means? I didn't, so I looked it up. (Of course, I did! I'm a writer, right?) According to one dictionary, it means "to withdraw companionship, protection, or support from somebody; to give up, renounce, or sacrifice something that gives pleasure".[12]

Guess what! You are God's companion (Don't you love that song, *I Am a Friend of God*[13]?), and He will not withdraw any of His blessing, His passion, or His protection from you. He will not sacrifice you. (He took care of that for us!) He will never forsake you.

Rest well tonight, my wonderful mother and friend, for you sit in the perfection of His love, and you bring Him great pleasure. As you bring to so many of us! Love you!

Carie

Thursday, April 3 —
Knowing God Is in Control of What Looks Like a Mistake

A quick update: My preparation for chemotherapy continues. I still have almost a week before I begin treatment, and God is bringing me to a place of trust in Him that is deeper than I have walked before. I am confident I will be ready by next week.

Monday morning, Charlie and I drove into Dallas to Presbyterian Heart Clinic for my heart sonogram. After waiting for some time to see the doctor, we discovered that communication had been mixed up and I was only scheduled for a consultation rather than a sonogram.

The doctor was very gracious. He called my oncologist and talked at length about what I needed. Then he explained things to us in detail and in a way that we could easily understand. What a gift. He ended up referring me to an associate whose office is in McKinney. She actually begins working there this week, and her office is in the same building as my oncologist. That will be an hour closer and more convenient than driving into Dallas. The associate doctor is a heart-muscle specialist, which will be a great asset in her monitoring my heart during the 5–6 months of treatment. I am blessed to see God work things out, even when they originally seemed to "not be working out!"

Because I didn't have the heart tests on Monday, Charlie and I took advantage of the extra time and of the rare privilege of being in Dallas, and we spent the rest of the day "playing." It was a fun day. We went to lunch and to Half Price Books and then took dinner to Charlie's mother and spent time with her.

The heart sonogram was rescheduled for Wednesday, so yesterday morning, I had an appointment with the oncologist at 10 a.m. to discuss the results of the tests I subsequently had at noon! Sounds like confusion but made us laugh. My appointment with the oncologist was short and good, as he answered questions I've had. The sonogram went well. I have another appointment with the oncologist next Monday morning to discuss the results of the tests. Those results will determine what treatment I start on Tuesday.

That is the practical report of the past few days. Thank you for your prayers. It is nice to rest in Him and trust that He is guiding our steps. Keeps the blood pressure down, too!

Saturday, April 5 — Being Prepared

The last morning I was in Japan in February, as I was packing and getting ready to go to the airport to return home, the Lord began to speak to me. I had just finished speaking at a ladies' conference and I was praising Him for all He did in the women's lives. I was praying for my family, for a safe trip home, and for my upcoming surgery, which was scheduled for three days after I returned home. God's words came to me with such great intensity that I had to stop and write down the things He was speaking so I would not forget or miss anything.

He spoke about "preparation." First, He instructed me to "be prepared." He said that "being prepared" is different from "getting prepared," and He gave me the following example. If Charlie told me to get dressed, that would mean one thing. But if Charlie told me to "be dressed," that would mean to not only *get* dressed but to *stay* dressed until he came for me or told me otherwise. *"Be prepared" is a condition of readiness.* I think the military calls it "mobilization readiness."

The Lord reminded me that He spoke to His Church before the turn of the century and told us to "be ready." Instead, we "got ready" for the things we thought might happen as the year 2000 began. When things didn't happen the way we thought and we saw no trauma or problems, we went back to our lives as they had been before. The stored water, prepared food, generators, and other emergency preparations were sold or given away.

For the past two months, my time has been focused on preparation — physical, mental, emotional, and spiritual — for the process that lies ahead, and all of that preparation has been very practical. I had to relinquish responsibilities, which is not easy for me. Admitting my limitations has been humbling, and some days requires more courage and greater faith than I think I have.

This week, I talked to a lady about cleaning my house for the next few months while I have treatment. Getting help is not something I ever wanted, but I know the help is necessary. It is one thing to quit activities because I don't have strength or feel well, but to stop when I feel great and have energy is a matter of obedience, and takes confidence that I am hearing the Lord. (I can't imagine Noah obeying God and building an ark when it had never rained before! He certainly had to know God's voice. See Genesis 6.)

When the doctor recommended that I have chemotherapy, he also said that one side effect of the particular drugs would be hair loss. As I have shared, I began preparing by having my hair cut very short. Then I went to the wig store, found the right wig, and ordered it. When it came in, I went back and had it styled. Then I began wearing it to church. When one friend discovered that my new hairdo was a wig, she asked me why I was already wearing it. I knew that if I waited until my hair fell out to begin to adjust, I would struggle with my emotions. It has been easier to adjust to wearing my wig and to learn how to take care of it while I feel strong physically and while my emotions are calm. The Lord keeps telling me to "be prepared."

In the past two weeks, I have read through all the information that the oncologist gave me concerning chemotherapy. That has not been easy. However, it was easier and less emotional this time than it was when I first received the information. I have the grace and strength to sort through the information and consume only what I need to know for the next step. I was finally able to do this without being emotionally overwhelmed.

Besides the emotional and practical preparations, I have also dealt with fears and doubts concerning chemotherapy. The Lord continues to reassure me of His presence—that He is not just "with me" but "in me." He has promised to guide all that happens in my body and to protect me. And He continues to tell me to "fear not."

I don't pretend to understand the impact or value of all God is saying. I just know *what* He is telling me. He reminded me of the parable of the 10 virgins (Matthew 25:1–13). Five were foolish and five were wise. The wise ones were those who prepared ahead of time and stayed ready for the bridegroom to come.

As the coming months unfold and I finish treatment, I will be interested to know what God wants me to do to "remain ready." I am confident that what I am walking through and what He is teaching me is not only for my present situation but also for my future. I am crying out to God to speak to His bride around the world and to help us *be* ready, *be* watchful, *be* alert, *be* clothed in armor, have our spiritual weapons sharpened, and to *be* prepared for His coming (Revelation 19:7). This preparation involves having patience and being faithful in investing our time and talents wisely until He comes. Sometimes, preparation involves fighting battles and standing against all that comes to steal the blessings, promises, and peace of God.

For me, being ready requires perseverance. There are many things I would rather do than prepare for chemotherapy. I would prefer to have fun, work in the pastures, paint my closet, continue living a "normal life" and ignore what is coming. But I know that would not be wise, and, with the Lord drawing me forward, I have sought to stay on course. I find my determination growing, sort of like the buffalo that, when the storm comes, turns *into* the storm knowing that as he moves head-on into the winds, he will get through it faster than if he stood still or ran from it. As I press forward, I find that the fear diminishes a little more each day.

I don't take for granted your prayers on my behalf. It takes an army to fight some battles and I could not fight this one by myself. I believe that the peace and strength, and even my ability to hear God and do what He tells me to do, are results of your prayers. I love and appreciate you for that gift. I remain very grateful as I prepare for the coming days and for what I do not know but what God does know!

❧ GUEST

Every time you send a journal entry, I am touched by the practical advice that applies to people everywhere. Thank you for listening to the Holy Spirit and for sharing those pertinent truths you are learning. I pass them on to others who are eager to hear the next update because of circumstances in their own lives and just because they are spiritually hungry.

Being prepared is something the Holy Spirit is speaking to me as well. Part of that, for me, is to arrive at places early rather than at the last minute. I am surprised that by being early, I am more peaceful, and instead of wasting time just waiting, I am available, even prepared, for "unexpected" opportunities to help others.

Having the grace to do what you must do at the appointed time speaks to me also. Many times I have declined to do something because I thought I could not, without realizing that God's grace and provision would be there when I needed it.

So I trust Him to protect you as only His love and power can in your body, soul, and spirit. Knowing that we are an army and not working alone fighting this battle is encouraging.

I love and appreciate you.
Dianna

Monday, April 7 — Being Prepared for Chemotherapy

This morning, I had an appointment with the oncologist to review the results of last week's heart tests. Because my heart is weak, the doctor recommended that my treatment include an additional medication that will protect my heart from some of the other chemicals. Carie was with me and understood all he said (what a blessing). She responded, "Mom, this is a good thing, a very wise decision . . . and an answer to my prayers!" That was encouragement!

My treatment will begin at 10 a.m. However, because my treatment includes additional medication, the oncologist will give me the entire treatment more quickly than originally planned. So instead of being in the office for five hours, I should be finished in three or four hours.

In my last journal entry, I wrote about some of the things the Lord has led me to do to "be prepared." But the other part is all that the Lord is doing to prepare me, even when I'm not aware that He's at work. He knows the future and has good plans for us (Jeremiah 29:11). We don't know what is ahead. But He is continually guiding our lives with His wisdom and love. Sometimes we have the privilege of seeing some of what He is doing.

About 16 months ago, I was at a luncheon with a group of ladies. We were asked to share what we wanted to accomplish, both spiritually and practically, in the coming year. I felt like my spiritual life and ministry were at a total standstill. I had no direction or vision for the coming year. I knew the Lord was working in me, but I felt stripped and empty, and it was *NOT* comfortable.

One of the ladies began explaining that eagles go to the top of the mountain and "molt" — lose all their feathers. The feathers gradually begin to grow back. The eagle can do nothing but wait for the process to be completed. Once the eagle has its "new coat," it is stronger and can fly higher than it ever did before. She said God had told her that I was like that eagle, and that this season was preparation. He would restore ministry to me, and I would be stronger and accomplish far more than before. She said this process was necessary equipping for my future.

The Lord does things in such divine and marvelous ways. (The world calls this "coincidence.") A few weeks ago, a friend sent the following encouragement to me. As I read it, I cried (of course) and then remembered those words spoken months ago. I began to rejoice at how graciously God has prepared me for "such a time as this" (Esther 4:14 NASB). Truly, He who knows all things, including the future, is faithful. And He is with us, working in and through us to bring about His plans.

EAGLES IN A STORM

Did you know that an eagle knows when a storm is approaching long before the storm breaks? The eagle will fly to some high spot and wait for the winds to come. When the storm hits, it sets its wings so that the wind will pick it up and lift it above the storm. While the storm rages below, the eagle is soaring above it. The eagle does not escape the storm. It simply uses the storm to lift it higher. It rises on the winds that bring the storm.

When the storms of life come upon us — and all of us will experience them — we can rise above them by setting our minds and our belief toward God. The storms do not have to overcome us. We can allow God's power to lift us above them. God enables us to ride the winds of the storm that brings sickness, tragedy, failure and disappointment in our lives. We can soar above the storm.

Remember, it is not the burdens of life that weigh us down, it is how we handle them.[14]

I wrote the above "eagle part" of this journal entry yesterday but did not post it. This morning, I received an email from a friend. She ended her message by saying, "*Soar like the eagle; let my encouragement be like the wind that keeps you high enough to fly without effort*" (Lissa).

Okay, I get it. God is speaking to me through so many of you, and I'm listening! Thank you for your obedience; thank you for your words of life and encouragement; thank you for being part of the "preparation process" in my life. And I thank Him for using you to speak to me!

The past few weeks have been intense, and I have continually bared my soul before the Lord. He has listened and has done such a deep work in me that today I have no fear. That *is* a *huge* miracle. Two weeks ago, I wanted to run away and never hear the word "chemotherapy" again.

Tomorrow is the beginning of a new season. I am ready and have strength and a tenacity that I have never experienced before. I have actually celebrated all day today as I have walked, once again, in His incredible peace.

GUEST

Your latest journal entry was so insightful. The call to "be ready" makes so much sense. Thank you for sharing the truths that God is giving you.

"For the Lord God will help me; therefore shall I not be confounded: therefore have I set my face like a flint, and I know that I shall not be ashamed" (Isaiah 50:7 KJV).

Tomorrow find that safe place with Jesus, and your prayer warriors will be in your shield.

Love you bunches,
Joyce

Thank you for sharing the words God has given you and for sharing with understanding and the testimony of your life. The peace God has given you far exceeds human reasoning and resources. As you walk this path, you are installing lights along the path so others can see how and where to walk. It dispels the darkness and fear.

As I imagine what it would be like to walk in your shoes, I can see the fear that I would experience. However, as you share your walk with me, I, too, can overcome them.

Your message of "being ready" and "staying ready" is truly a word for me today. I will hold fast those words in my heart.

With gratitude for who you are in Christ.

Love,
Abigale

Tuesday, April 8 — Taking the First Chemotherapy Treatment

I am home after treatment and am doing very well. I was not prepared to feel so good, but I was told that it takes time for the drugs to begin to do their job, and then the side effects normally set in. I am tired. I just took a nap and could go to bed for the evening. Instead, I am getting ready to eat dinner and watch a basketball game with Charlie . . . at least until I fall asleep!

Thank you for your prayers. During the day, Charlie and I talked with every other patient in the infusion room. The treatment nurses were running about an hour late, so we were actually there for more than five hours. The nurses explained step by step what they were doing and what to watch for. I am grateful to be this far along.

🌾 GUEST

I trust God's presence there with you during treatments. I am comforted that you feel so well.

I'm finding as I read through the Old Testament again that God's promises are so amazing. His Word makes it plain: obedience reaps blessings; disobedience reaps curses. (I am glad He recognizes even my *efforts* to obey and that He is merciful when I miss the mark).

He is our Provision, our Shield, our Comforter, our High Tower, our Healer, our Ever Present Help, our Hope. . . . There is no good thing that He does not provide for His children. I like thinking of His glorious love and power, His nature, and His goodness toward us — what a mighty God!

Thankful,
Dianna

❧ GUEST

I was very nervous about seeing you undergo chemotherapy, but what a blessing: your amazing courage, your tenacity (that's our new word, isn't it?), and your willingness to reach out to those in the treatment room. Wonder what the Holy Spirit accomplished yesterday? Looks like a huge victory to me! And we claim that, right?

We don't know what you will experience today or tomorrow. I am praying that you are miraculously strong and encouraged and refreshed! I am praying that God will provide you with strength.

I was looking up names of God and found several I'd not seen before.

- He is Jehovah-Chatsahi (**Lord my Strength**): "The Lord is my light and my salvation — whom shall I fear? The Lord is the stronghold of my life — of whom shall I be afraid?" (Psalm 27:1).

- He is Jehovah-'Izoa Hakaboth (**Lord Strong and Mighty**): "Who is this King of glory? The Lord strong and mighty, the Lord mighty in battle" (Psalm 24:8).

- He is Jehovah-Tsori (**Lord my Strength and Shield**): "The Lord is my strength and my shield; my heart trusts in him, and I am helped. My heart leaps for joy and I will give thanks to him in song" (Psalm 28:7).

May you sense His strength today!

I love you!
Carie

Thursday, April 10 — Experiencing the Peace of God

I am so grateful to have had a smooth couple of days. I am learning to be more disciplined about eating, which makes a big difference. I have had very little nausea (yeah!), though I am very tired. I am living a fairly normal life but in slow motion. I had hoped to go to church last night, but about 3 p.m. I knew my energy was running low, and I was asleep by 8 p.m. I do feel like things are going well.

I thought back to what my friend Keri said — that "cancer picked the wrong person to mess with." The more I think about her statement, the more I realize that the enemy thought he was just picking on *me*, but instead he discovered that an army has been raised up to fight against him. Thank you as you help enforce Christ's victory in my life.

During the night last night, the Lord took me to a Scripture from Habakkuk 3:19 (AMP):

> The Lord God is my Strength, my personal bravery, and my invincible army; He makes my feet like hinds' feet and will make me to walk [not to stand still in terror, but to walk] and make [spiritual] progress upon my high places [of trouble, suffering, or responsibility]!

What an amazing miracle it is to continue walking in peace and not in fear. As Charlie and I went into the treatment room on Tuesday, we were able to focus on reaching out to others. We tried to encourage each person there and many of them encouraged us also.

God is faithful. I also thank each of you for your faithfulness to pray and encourage our family as we walk this journey. May He return many blessings to you as you have blessed us.

Saturday, April 12 — Fulfilling His Purposes

Being a career military man, Charlie has been a student of strategic and tactical warfare for many years. However, his greatest interest has been in the Civil War. He once told me how the opposing armies would line up facing each other and begin to fight, as we have often seen in movies. At times, civilians would sit on the hillsides, watching the battle. That describes where I am. I am observing a battle that is going on in my body. The chemotherapy has begun to work and I can feel it happening, but I can only sit and watch and wait. The medications are attacking the fast-growing cells. At the same time, my body is fighting to rebuild and protect itself. I am grateful that the One who made me (Psalm 139) and knows how many hairs are on my head (Matthew 10:30) is here inside me, refereeing and directing this match.

I am not a good spectator. I prefer to be involved in whatever is going on (except sporting events and garage sales, which I prefer to watch!), so I need to adjust and discipline myself. Imagine — discipline.

At the end of last year, the Lord told me that my most frequent prayer for the coming year would be to ask for patience. (Later I asked Him if He didn't mean "patients?") I now see that He is teaching me patience and endurance, and He says I am to ". . . let endurance have its perfect result, so that you may be perfect and complete, lacking in nothing" (James 1:4 NASB). Some versions say, ". . . let patience have her perfect work . . ." (James 1:4a KJV). I am grateful that He is using this journey to bring about eternal purposes and to refine and mold my character.

I do not want to simply count the days until treatment is over. I want each day to be used for His purposes. Because of personal experience, I can now pray for people in ways that I couldn't before. I am growing in compassion. I also have to spend time resting, so I can use that time to pray. I have an appreciation for life that has increased over the past few months. He is building precious things into my life through my circumstances, and I don't want to lose anything.

The key for me is to keep my eyes on Him rather than on myself. I can easily focus on "me" — on how I feel, what hurts, what I want or don't want. If the Lord leads you to pray for me, please pray that I will keep my focus on Jesus, "the author and perfecter of [my] faith . . ." (Hebrews 12:2 NASB). That is the place of peace, joy, blessing, and gratitude. I have experienced the difference and know how I want to live!

Thank you for walking with me! You make a difference in my life and the life of my family.

❧ GUEST

It is good to know that You are Almighty God. You aren't just mighty — You are might and You are more powerful than anything else that exists.

I pray that You would be mighty in Mom's body today. Thank You for her courage to surrender all to You. Thank You that because You are faithful to Your children, You will not allow her to walk through this without Your grace and healing touch, and You will not ask her to go through anything she cannot handle in Your power.

Please help her body to heal supernaturally. Thank You that, as You allow chemotherapy to purge her body of unwanted cells, Your Spirit continues to challenge and grow her so she can further spread Your love and Your truth on this earth.

Bless her, and please bless those who faithfully pray for her and for Daddy and for our family. Please protect Mom and Dad and keep them sheltered in You. Amen.

Love you, Mom (and Daddy). Hope today was refreshment and encouragement. The children send their love — they all miss you a lot.

Carie

❧ GUEST

Thanks . . . for writing . . . about warfare strategies. . . . I recently read an urgent prayer request from Dutch Sheets . . . and he referred to World War II prayer strategies that changed the outcome . . . also we have the book by Derek Prince on changing history through prayer and fasting. We will keep in mind how God continually answered the prayers of the righteous! Thanks for reminding us that the Lord is first and foremost even in and especially in battle.

Love,
Darleen

Tuesday, April 15—Warrior Cells and Present Faith

Yesterday, I went to the oncologist's office for lab work. The weekend was a physical challenge, but by Monday morning, I felt better. The doctor decided to give me a shot to boost my white blood cells (WBCs). I was told to expect a lot of pain for a few days after the shot. I am grateful that so far I have had none.

After my appointment, I went to lunch with Carie and her children. Sitting at lunch, Elisabeth gave me a medical lesson, telling me some amazing things. I am the most "unmedical" person I know, so in the past few months I have heard more medical terms than I ever hoped to hear. And I remember very few of them. I do know a few basic words, like surgery. And I know that the chemotherapy is a "T," an "A," and a "C" drug: the "TAC" formula. I tried to remember the names and quickly forgot them. I figure as long as the doctor remembers what I need and I write information down in case I need to know, that is enough for me.

Carie explained to me about red blood cells, which was fascinating. (I saw a movie about that once . . . people being shrunk and journeying through the body. I remember that the blood cells looked really big to them!)

Then Elisabeth announced that I had just received an injection of "warriors cells" that were going to fight for me! There was tremendous encouragement in her statement. I have warriors on the "outside," prayer warriors who are fighting for me. Now I have "warriors" on the inside fighting for me also. Who can beat that?

I keep saying, "I am taking one day at a time," which sounds so silly, as if it is possible for anyone to live any other way! One day, even one minute at a time, is all there is. We only have the "now moment."

Two weeks ago, Charlie taught at church on "present faith." He used the example of Mary and Martha when Lazarus died (John 11). "Martha said to Jesus, 'Lord, if you had been here, my brother would not have died'" (John 11:21 NKJV). They had *past faith*. Then, when Jesus asked if they believed in the resurrection, they turned to the future and acknowledged that "in the last day" there will be a resurrection (v. 24). They had *future faith*. But, Jesus wanted them to have "*present faith*" and trust Him for what was needed that moment.

This moment is all that I have and I want to make the most of it. I want present faith for what I am walking through *now*. Present faith brings the Kingdom of Heaven into my life and makes it a reality.

Thank you again, prayer warriors, for fighting for me and for blessing our lives.

✣ GUEST

These journal entries are too good for this scenario not to be planned by a loving Father. The Lord had this all thought out and just needed your cooperation. You are on stage with words appropriate for many people in many situations about walking by faith, and the audience is growing. That is grace in action. You allow us to see you when you are weak, leaving yourself transparent. You are taking us with you on this journey, and are giving out spiritual nuggets that you are taking in.

Thank you for your sense of humor—my medical knowledge is right up there with yours! The warrior illustration, outside and in, is encouraging.

Thankful with you for God's goodness and His presence, with love,

Dianna

✣ GUEST

Just keep on believing, trusting, receiving, knowing. . . . God is on the throne and He is in control. Nothing that is happening in you (or in any of us) takes Him by surprise, and He is not shaken by it. I am so thankful that we can trust Him with every situation and know that He is working for our ultimate good and His glory.

Thank you for allowing Him to be glorified in your life and for sharing that journey with those who care for you and love you.

Darlene

✣ GUEST

Mom, did you know that a group of men now make up the "new" Imperials? I heard them sing an oldie but goodie yesterday on the radio. It brought back lots of memories, but I thought it was just as appropriate for today as it was—wow—30 years ago. . . .

When you're up against a struggle that shatters all
        your dreams
And your hope's been cruelly crushed by Satan's
        manifested scheme
And you feel the urge within you to submit to earthly
        fears
Don't let the faith you're standing in seem to
        disappear.

Praise the Lord—He can work through those who
        praise Him
Praise the Lord—for our God inhabits praise
Praise the Lord—for the chains that seem to bind you
        serve only to remind you that they drop
        powerless behind you when you praise Him.[15]

Love you and am praising God for His power in you!

Christie

Thursday, April 17 — Timetable for Chemotherapy

Today, I visited the oncologist's office again for lab work. My WBCs, "warrior cells," seem to have battle fatigue, so the doctor put me on antibiotics. I feel great; I just can't keep my eyes open!

Several people have asked about my schedule. Charlie says the doctor has a "matrix," which means there is a list of things that have to line up in my body before I have another chemotherapy treatment. It has to do with WBC count and also with the results of the heart sonograms that I have between each treatment. (I go to "nuclear medicine" for this test. The men who work there are wonderful, and they make Charlie and me laugh.) When the numbers all line up properly, then I will have the next treatment.

At present, the treatments are set for every three weeks on Tuesdays. We initially set the date for the second treatment so I would be at maximum strength to minister at a women's conference in Ruidoso, New Mexico, the last weekend in April. I will speak on the subject of "Preparing the Bride of Christ." I am scheduled to speak Friday evening, Saturday morning, Saturday evening. On Sunday morning, I will give a brief conclusion and serve communion. Carie is going with me to drive and to take care of me.

If all goes according to the "matrix," I will have my second treatment on April 29, right after returning from New Mexico.

I am very aware that often when we set up "expectations" and they don't come about as we think they should or want them to, it opens a door for disappointment. *God does not disappoint*; only my own plans and expectations bring disappointment. I am seeking to walk in that "present faith" for today and know that God has His own timetable for my life. His timetable was written before I was born (Psalm 139:16). His plan is good, not for evil (Jeremiah 29:11–13). And none of what I am facing is too difficult for Him (Jeremiah 32:17). I don't want to limit what He is doing by setting my heart on a particular timetable, so I am not yet planning a party for the end of the summer. But I do promise that whenever this is over, I *will* have a party!

I am so thankful that when the "inner warriors" are taking a rest, many of you continue to pray and support me. *Thank you so much*! You truly demonstrate the love of God to my life.

❧ GUEST

This morning, the children and I read 2 Chronicles 14. Asa was king of Judah; he obeyed God and had 10 years of peace. Then the Ethiopians came against Judah and outnumbered Judah, two to one. Asa prayed, "Lord, there is no one besides Thee to help in the battle between the powerful and those who have no strength; so help us, O Lord our God, for we trust in Thee, and in Thy name have come against this multitude. O Lord, Thou art our God; let not man prevail against Thee" (2 Chronicles 14:11 NASB).

Then I read your warrior entry and this is the prayer I will pray for you today, "We trust in Thee, Lord; let not disease or this treatment prevail against Thee."

May the Lord multiply your "warriors" and may His hand defeat any disease that comes against you as you make this pro-life statement and as you share your spiritual life through this website.

Onward, soldier! :-) Love you and Daddy!

Carie

GUEST

Thank you, again, for taking the time and energy to bring us into your path of experience. Whatever the outward circumstances, many of us will face medical situations that require us to stand by faith and not by sight, to be patient and to trust God to act according to His timetable. Realizing that it is my own expectations that disappoint me and not God's plans for me (His plans are always for good) — puts a perspective on life and on situations that allows my faith to remain steady. Thank you for encouraging me again.

I am grateful for the steadfast love and attention of Charlie to help, and for your children and grandchildren who surround you and love you. Mostly, I am thankful for the obvious work of the Holy Spirit on a daily basis in your life — Jesus sticking closer than a brother (Proverbs 18:24). What is coming out of that relationship is teaching and blessing the rest of us who are marching around you. God is good!

> With love and prayers,
> Dianna

GUEST

Good morning Suzanne! I hope that you are enjoying the sunshine and wonderful weather. I was working in my garden and had a wonderful thing happen. I turned over a large decorative rock to find thousands of little ants and thousands of their little white eggs. Immediately the ants instinctively stopped everything and began taking each egg to a safe place so it would survive. Those little ants didn't have a "big" ant telling them what to do. I didn't hear a horn or see screens come up with instructions. They just knew what their job was and did it. I watched for the next few minutes as they carefully rescued every single white egg from that side of the rock.

OK, this has to be a picture of how those warrior WBCs are being protected and cared for by our loving Father and the very plan for health to be restored to your body. As I watched the ants, I remembered the parable about the ants — "Go to the ant . . . observe her ways and be wise, which having no chief, officer, or ruler, prepares her food in the summer, and gathers her provision in the harvest" (Proverbs 6:6–8 NASB). Ants just do what they are intended to do — it's their mission. And they have provision in the harvest. So it is with those WBCs in your body. They don't need to be told what to do; they just do it! It's their mission. They busily go about their job and when you need the harvest of healing, it's there. I may be simplifying, but that was a great picture of the success of little tiny creations of God that aren't necessarily strong (couldn't move the rock), but they certainly get their job done!

I had a great time praying for your WBCs as a result of my little ant experience and believe it is just as evident in your body right now. God is always so obvious in His creation, and I truly enjoyed seeing how He's caring for everything that will fight for you. There's a plan, Suzanne, for your healing, restoration, and redemption of this entire matter so that you shine more brightly than before and bless others with expanded wisdom and power. Praise God. May your WBCs do all they are intended and may they "bite" anything that tries to prevent it! It's a beautiful day.

Much love,
Susan T.

Monday, April 21 — Fearing the Known

Years ago, as a young officer, Charlie had a commander who taught him how to train the young military men and women who worked for him. The commander, a general, said, "If you pour gasoline into a glass, when you shake the glass, gasoline comes out. Likewise, whatever you pour into those young men and women is what will come out of them when they are shaken."

Often we think "shaking" (i.e., "trials") is bad. But I am learning that when things are going smoothly, I don't really know what my character is like. I can even fool myself into thinking I am very "spiritual." It is during those times when my life is shaken that I discover what is inside.

Over the past few months, I have discovered that there are some good solid truths deeply rooted in my life. I get excited and am sometimes surprised when those good things come out. However, there are also some things coming out of my life that are not so Godly. I am becoming very grateful when those attitudes and actions surface. It's not that I'm happy that they are in my life, but that God cares enough to make me aware of things that are not pleasing to Him. And He does that to clean them out of my life.

Many times, I have heard Charlie teach, "When God shows you sin and weaknesses in your life, *it is not for your condemnation or discouragement but is for your encouragement.* God is saying that you don't have to stay that way. He is making you aware of those things so He can clean them out of your life." So, today I am grateful for revelation, for the deeper things of the Lord I am learning, and for awareness of things inside me that need to be cleaned out.

Last summer, a friend prayed over the issue of "dread" in my heart. I was not aware of any dread in my life. But when she prayed, I not only knew it was true, I knew that God was hearing her prayer and was cleaning it out of my heart. The result was peace and freedom. Dread is a form of fear: "To fear greatly; be in extreme apprehension of; to be reluctant to do, meet, or experience".[16] I have dealt with layers of fear in my life and have made progress, but this was another layer.

As I face the second chemotherapy treatment, which is a week away, I have apprehension and reluctance. The fear I dealt with before the first treatment two weeks ago (seems like two months ago) was fear of the "unknown." Now I find that the issue is fear of the "known." In the past two days, I have finally felt good—almost normal. And last night, I had my first night of sleep with no pain and no pain medication since the treatment. I have been told that the effects of the treatments are accumulative: the more chemotherapy you have, the more extreme the side effects tend to be. Yesterday, I realized I dread having to start the process all over again. So, last night I got serious about dealing with it.

The peace came when I was studying the word "hope." Hope means "favorable and confident expectation".[17]

I do not look forward to the physical effects of chemotherapy, so how do I reconcile that with hope? Sometimes the facts of our situations seem so overwhelming that we cannot imagine expecting anything good, much less "confident and favorable expectation." I am faced once again with the understanding that I have the ability to choose where I focus my attention. When I focus on my circumstances, I begin to dread. That dread leads to thoughts of painful possibilities, and I experience a snowball effect of discouragement, anxiety, and depression. Self-focus has the potential to kill, steal, and destroy all that I am created to do and to be.

God-focus—remembering who God is, what He has done, all He has promised to do—builds my hope. In fact, my hope then tends to increase—

to snowball — and as it does, I am filled with peace, joy, and gratitude. I know where to find life, and it is not in dread. Life is in Jesus who alone *is* Life (John 14:6).

My hope can only be established in the Lord and in His presence. He says hope is the ". . . anchor of the soul . . . which enters within the veil" (Hebrews 6:19 NASB). That means hope is connected deep in my soul and firmly attached (anchored) to His presence. The veil was the curtain in the Old Testament tabernacle that separated the people from the presence of God. That veil was literally and supernaturally ripped apart when Jesus died on the cross (Matthew 27:50–51). Through Jesus, we have access to the living God (Hebrews 10:19-20). He is the source and object of our hope, not only in the afterlife but also here on earth where for us as Christians, eternal life begins.

So, as I prepare for next week, I am praying for hope to be deeply established in my soul. I pray that my focus will not be dread of pain, sleeplessness, or other side effects, but that I will have confident expectation in His eternal purposes. I desire for God to work in and through me and do miracles daily as He has promised.

⅊ GUEST

I just read your latest entry and wanted to pass something along that I wrote years ago. After doing a word study on the Hebrew root for "encouragement," I wrote the following:

> **Encouragement:** To fasten upon God's grace and mercy. To be strong in the power of His love. To be courageous in heart. To strengthen your weak knees. To cure the trembling hands. To help the fainting soul. To repair the broken places. To fortify the weaker areas. To conquer your fears. To mend relationships. To cleave to God's faithfulness. To confirm your beliefs. To be constant in the Holy Spirit. To constrain your emotions. To continue the race. To be of good courage. To encourage yourself in God's Word. To be established in Jesus. To withstand the attack. To harden yourself against the enemy. To help yourself by trusting. To lay hold and hold fast to truth. To lean on God's understanding. To maintain peace. To mend your torn soul. To wax mighty by God's power. To prevail over

principalities. To be recovered by the cross. To retain God's knowledge. To strengthen yourself. To be stout and not shaken. To take hold of truth. To valiantly behave yourself.

Continuing to lift you up in prayer to the Father,

Lana

Thursday, April 24 — Losing My Hair and Hearing God's Voice

Tuesday was a day I anticipated ever since I heard the word "chemotherapy." From the beginning, the Lord showed me that I would have to go through every step of the process of healing. The Lord said that Tuesday was the day for me to have my hair cut off, so I made an appointment and Charlie planned to go with me.

I have shared with you how I began to prepare by finding and purchasing my wig. I immediately began wearing my "new hair" to get used to it. I went through a period of grief over the idea of losing my hair but quickly settled the issue in my heart as I came to the obvious realization that hair has no eternal value. I am more than my hair, and it will eventually grow back. Carie even told me that losing my hair is a good sign, because it is proof that the chemotherapy is doing what it is intended to do — killing off all fast-growing cells.

I believe that every step is part of the equipping God is placing in my life to more effectively minister to others, and I know He is using this experience to draw me into a deeper trust and intimacy with Him.

He had impressed on my heart that if I had my hair cut on Tuesday, I would be free to focus on ministering to the ladies at the retreat this weekend rather than thinking about my shedding hair. However, as I approached Tuesday, I struggled inside. I kept going back to the Lord and asking if He really meant for me to do this. I didn't want to be disobedient. I checked my heart to see if it was self-pity. I kept wondering why I was having a difficult time because I thought I had dealt with the issue.

The main reason I struggled was because my hair wasn't falling out. I wondered, "What if by some strange reason my hair doesn't fall out and I go cut it off for no reason?" Several people, out of their love and concern for me, had tried to encourage me that my hair would not fall out. But I began to listen to what *they* said instead of what *God* had said, and it brought confusion. I lost my focus.

Finally, on Monday night, I was tired of the turmoil and I began crying out to the Lord. I told Him that if I had my hair cut and it didn't fall out, I was going to be very upset! But, I finally said, "Lord, I am going to do what I believe You have told me to do. My hair will get cut off tomorrow. If I am missing You and Your plan, please show me because I want to be obedient. I am going to trust that I have heard from You."

Shortly after that prayer, I reached up to touch my hair and a large clump of hair fell out in my hand. I wondered if God was watching me and smiling, saying, "Just watch what I am going to do for my daughter, Suzanne. I know exactly what she needs and when she needs it!"

I got *so* excited that I ran upstairs yelling, "My hair is falling out!" Charlie was stunned and sat looking at me, not sure what to say. Then I said, "I am so thankful! I *can* hear from God!" I explained to Charlie how I had struggled all day. The issue was not my hair. The real issue was *being able to hear God's voice.* That is often the bottom line. When I hear from God, I know all will be well and He will take care of things. But when I doubt my ability to hear His voice or know His will, I am open to confusion and unbelief.

Tuesday, I had my hair cut and I was full of peace. My heart was set on obeying God, reaching out to others, and not focusing on myself. I am very thankful that I will not be shedding this weekend at the retreat. And I will not be distracted, but I can focus on the ladies and their needs.

While I was having my hair cut, Charlie and I had the opportunity to minister to the man who cut my hair and who had sold me my wig. Recently, two employees left his business and started a competing business. He was very discouraged. We were able to encourage him and prayed for the prosperity of His business and ministry. He was obviously blessed and very grateful. We expect God to continue to do good things through his business.

Hearing God's voice is a major issue in the life of a Christian. Christianity *is* personal relationship with the living God. Relationship involves two-way communication. Jesus said, "My sheep hear my voice . . ." (John 10:27 NASB).

I had no problems hearing God's voice as I worked on four teachings for the retreat in New Mexico. But when it came to the personal and emotional issue of my hair, I had problems knowing I was hearing Him, especially when I began listening to voices that spoke contrary to what God had already said. What a blessing to know that even during times of confusion and doubt, God will speak to us. He cares, and He is willing to speak in such a way that we recognize His voice.

When God told Abraham to sacrifice his son, Isaac (Genesis 22:1–14), Abraham was totally confident that he was hearing God. It was through Isaac that all God's promises to Abraham and his descendants — the Jewish nation — were to be fulfilled. Yet, when God said, "Offer Isaac as a sacrifice," *Abraham was willing to trust God rather than his own ideas or emotions.* When God saw the extent of Abraham's obedience, God provided a ram for the sacrifice, and God's name is revealed as Jehovah Jireh — "God will provide." He *is* our provision. Abraham's obedience was counted to Him as righteousness and was called "faith." In Hebrews 11:17–19, we read that Abraham was willing to offer up Isaac because He believed "God is able to raise people even from the dead . . ." (Hebrews 11:19a NASB). Abraham knew God so well that he knew if Isaac became the burnt offering, God would bring Isaac back to life and fulfill His promise. At that time in history, there is no indication that anyone had been raised from the dead. God had to have revealed this to Abraham beforehand. Oh, for such faith, and to know we hear God's voice so clearly!

Mine was certainly not a life-or-death situation, but even in this small matter, God was faithful to reassure me of my ability to hear His voice.

I have been told that I will have this short hair for several days until all of my hair is gone. And until it grows out again next fall, "Peaches" the wig is easy and convenient, and I am grateful for the provision.

Carie and I leave tomorrow morning for New Mexico. I am thankful for the opportunity to minister, and we are both very excited about going together. This will be my first time to minister to military women in the U.S. instead of overseas, and the first time for me and Carie to minister together. This is the fulfillment of desires I have had for years.

Please pray for the Lord's faithfulness to touch and change lives. Also, please pray for Charlie and Carie's family as they are home without us. Thank you again for continuing to bless our lives.

❧ GUEST

Know that you are being lifted up in prayer these days! I feel very close to you through your updates on this website, and that is a privilege. God's heart and perspective on life are always fascinating to me. I think "Oh, now I've got it, He really thinks outside the box." And then I get another insight, and start all over. . . . "Wow, God really thinks outside the box." That's what your perspective did today for me! He knows the number of the hairs on our head, whether they are home grown or imported!

Love,
Polly

GUEST

I was thinking about you Tuesday, knowing that your hair would be falling out about then. Did you ever think you would be excited about your hair falling out? I smiled when I read that. God certainly provides and His timing is always perfect!

I'm sure you look beautiful in your pixie cut. Here's a tip— adhesive tape works well when you get down to the last bit of hair and you want it to come on out (haha!).

Can't wait to see Peaches!

Love,
Susan

GUEST

You previously mentioned getting your hair cut as part of your preparation before chemotherapy. And now, you have completed another step of preparation in the ongoing process of healing by having your hair cut again so you don't have to deal with handfuls of hair as it falls out.

I recall that you have said that God takes you through each step of the teaching He wants to give through you. You are teaching on "Preparation of the Bride." Although having your hair fall out does not appear in the natural to be preparation a bride would want to make before her wedding, your obedience is preparation in the spiritual realm for what God has in mind for you.

You wrote that this is the first time for you to minister to military women in the U.S., and that this was a fulfillment of a desire you've had for years. I love God's ways. . . . I am so excited to see God's affirmation that He is doing a new thing and you will see it happen (Isaiah 43:19). I praise God for what I see Him doing in you, and I am blessed by your response to His way of doing things. What a privilege to be part of your life!

I love you!
Linda

Saturday, April 26 — Being Strengthened for Ministry

Carie and I are in New Mexico, and the ladies' retreat has already been amazing. The needs cover a vast spectrum, and many of the women have deep hurts. The group includes six teenagers and three young mothers who brought their new babies. God is at work. Thank you for your prayers. Tonight is a night for deep work. Only the Lord can minister to each person here.

I am feeling good. I have strength and slept well last night. I am grateful. I know the Lord is sustaining me and your prayers are upholding me. You are a valuable part of what is happening here.

Monday, April 28 — Coming Home Bald

Carie and I arrived home from New Mexico about 10:00 p.m. last night. This is Carie's last week of classes for this semester. She has several projects and a final exam to complete the requirements for her master's degree in technical communication. She is also teaching two undergraduate classes and has projects and a final exam to grade. I was so grateful to have her with me in New Mexico but also amazed that, in the midst of her pressing schedule, she would give her time to go with me.

The Lord used Carie to minister to the ladies. She encouraged them and prayed for many of them. Also, as one of you said, the unity and love between Carie and me was an encouragement, especially to the mothers.

I was privileged to minister this weekend. One of the teenagers said she heard God speak to her for the first time as I ministered on Saturday night. That was major breakthrough for this young woman, who is in the middle of tremendous turmoil in her life. These women needed physical healing, healing in marriages, healing in hearts, and encouragement.

God gave me practical teachings, and one lady said I had answered questions she'd had for years about the sovereignty of God. Another lady told me that she was in a spiritual battle, but she had never heard the word "intercession" before. She wanted to know more. As she explained her situation, I realized how ill equipped she felt but also saw how God is leading her one step at a time. Much work was done in lives, but those ladies will continue to be in my heart and prayers for a long time to come. Thank you for your prayers. The Lord answered abundantly.

I had energy and strength for each session. I slept both nights and was able to get a nap on Saturday afternoon. I was exhausted by the time I got home but had strength for all I needed to do.

Early tomorrow morning, I am scheduled for blood tests and for an appointment with the oncologist to review last week's heart scan. If all is in order, I will have the second chemotherapy treatment at 10 a.m. I am not fearful and have no dread. I am ready.

I spent today unpacking, doing laundry, grocery shopping, getting some meals ready for the next few days, and getting the rest of my "short hair" completely cut off. It was shedding and I was glad to have it gone. (What a miracle!) I have to laugh, as the reason I was ready — and glad — was because I didn't want hair all over my house! And what a precious thing it was to have Charlie look at me, in my almost bald state, and tell me how beautiful I am! True or not, I loved hearing him say it.

This journey gets more amazing each day. I thank the Lord for the reality of His presence, which I feel so powerfully. Nothing can shake that; nothing can compare with it. I am praying for opportunities to minister to someone tomorrow, someone who needs to know Him and have His presence in their life.

Again, thank you for your love, encouragement, and prayers. I can't imagine this walk without you!

Tuesday, April 29 — Facing Second Chemo Dread Free

Just a quick note to thank you for the prayers. I had my appointments this morning. My WBC count was back to normal, and the heart scan showed acceptable results, so I had the second treatment, which only lasted three hours. I am home and on my way to bed for a nap. Funny how I've not done anything but sit today and yet my body is exhausted!

Tomorrow, I return to the hospital to get the WBC-producer shot. Last time, I didn't get this shot until a week after chemotherapy. This time the oncologist wants to try to prevent the WBC count from dropping rather than having to build them up again with antibiotics. He says taking the shot early may cause me to have more pain. Last time, I did not react to the shot, which they say is rare — another miracle God has given to me! Taking the shot early may even prevent some of the reactions I had last time; I am trusting Him with all of this.

The treatment room was full this morning and I talked to most of the people having treatment. I am amazed at the joy and kindness of the people who work in the oncologist's office. Their work is truly a calling. They are so precious; I look forward to being with them.

Perhaps the greatest praise is that yesterday was a wonderful day — dread free! And today, when I woke up, I had no fear and no dread, and before I got out of bed, I was rejoicing that God had made this day for me. He will give me all that I need to walk victoriously. I knew many were praying; I could feel the strength. Thank you!

GUEST

You continue to be in our prayers, and we rejoice with you in the miracles God is working in and through you! You remind me of the Scripture in Joshua 1:8-9 (KJV):

> This book of the law shall not depart out of thy mouth; but thou shalt meditate therein day and night, that thou mayest observe to do according to all that is written therein: for then thou shalt make thy way prosperous, and then thou shalt have good success. Have not I commanded thee? Be strong and of a good courage; be not afraid, neither be thou dismayed: for the Lord thy God is with thee whithersoever thou goest.

I know you meditate on the Word constantly and are diligently persevering to obey God in every aspect of your life. It's evident that God is giving you daily courage and grace for the mission at hand. Those folks whom you meet at the oncologist's office (staff and patients) are so blessed and loved by God — to be ministered to and encouraged by God through you! What a powerful sermon your life preaches! I thank God for you!

Love you,
Delaine

Thursday, May 1 — Receiving Daily Manna

Yesterday, I felt great and full of energy. I have had no nausea with this treatment. I went to the oncologist's office for the WBC-booster shot and had no follow-up pain! I am thankful. Last time, the day after the treatment, I was in bed by 5:30 p.m., but last night I even had enough energy to go to church.

Today, I have less energy. My goal is to do laundry and to pick strawberries and sugar peas. Our garden is growing and must be tended every day. Now that I am picking sugar peas, I need to decide what to do with them. These are not the hard round yucky peas, but are sweet and delicious. We have an abundant crop.

I am increasingly aware that the joy of the Lord is my strength (Nehemiah 8:10), as I daily walk in joy. He has a plan for each day. I wake up praying for wisdom to know what He wants me to do and how to spend the strength He gives me. He will supply what I need. Being a good steward with my energy is a new area of discipline for me.

I have seen how talking takes much of my energy. So, this website continues to be a blessing because I can read and answer when I have the strength. It is difficult to express how precious and valuable your words are and how much they encourage me.

❧ GUEST

How remarkable is our God! He always gives testimony when we obey. The reasons for testimony are always different, but He definitely rewards obedience. I appreciate your example.

I agree that talking takes energy. I notice it too. Listening is easier, depending partly on who we are listening to. But listening to God brings my tensions to my attention because my facial muscles, which I did not notice were tight, suddenly relax. I am most at rest when I listen to Him. He arrests my anxieties! God is so loving and caring! Regardless of what is going on around me, in His presence, I am blessed. His presence is healthy! The song, "In His Presence," ministers to me: "In His presence, all fear is gone. . . . In His presence is where I belong".[18] That supersedes geographic location or the people around me.

I love you and am thankful for your testimonies.

Dianna

❧ GUEST

Be filled with trust and confidence in the Lord. Like a deeply rooted tree, you have no fear of the heat of chemotherapy—no worries of drought. Your leaves are always green and you never fail to bear fruit. May the sweet fruit of your lips (shared through your fingertips) bring encouragement and life to all who partake (based on Jeremiah 17:7–8 and Hebrews 13:15).

Love you,
Sarah

Friday, May 2 — Cultivating Peas and Bearing Fruit

Okay, I have to laugh about all the responses to "peas!" Our sugar peas are similar to Chinese snow peas. Charlie and I don't have them often because when I see how much they cost, I realize they are truly a delicacy. We steam them, put them in salads, or eat them raw as a snack. Someone suggested eating them in a sandwich. That sounds great—thanks. I suggest you try them. They truly redeem the concept of "peas!"

The signs of spring are everywhere. We have an abundance of redbirds and hummingbirds this spring. We have water in our tanks, which draws ducks, cranes, and turtles. The grass in the pastures is almost two feet tall. Charlie is outside mowing as I write. I can hear him singing and praying as he rides past by my window on the tractor.

The garden is growing. It's amazing to see how much it changes from day to day. The rain, the sun, the heat, and the cool weather all help the plants to grow and bear fruit. I guess God sees us sort of like that, as we receive the nutrition of His warmth, His Word, and His Spirit in our lives; together, it all brings growth. And then, we begin to blossom and bear fruit. It is exciting to see the parallels.

Today is one of those days of "heat" in my life. I have considerable pain, but though it may slow me down, it will not stop me. I am keeping a technical journal, and I noticed that several days after my last treatment, the pain began to affect what I could do. I am resting today from physical labor. Each day has different challenges and blessings. God is faithful. His presence is very near and real today, and I am grateful!

❧ GUEST

I always enjoy reading your journal entries. As I sometimes slip over the line and start to feel concern, which I suppose is a little okay, I gain this fantastic sense of peace realizing that you are in God's loving hands. It really does push me back into this wonderful place of peace. Thanks for sharing your ups and downs with us, and you are always on our minds and in our prayers.

We grow sugar peas, too, and they are great!

Love,
JB

❧ GUEST

My prayer is that today will be all that you need it to be. May the peace of God and the freshness of the Holy Spirit rest in your thoughts, rule in your dreams, and conquer all your fears. May God manifest himself today in ways you have never experienced, and may your joys be fulfilled, your dreams be closer, and your prayers be answered. I pray that faith enters a new height for you. I pray that your territory is enlarged. I pray for peace, healing, health, happiness, prosperity, joy, true and undying love for God. We love you and Charlie!

Pat

Sunday, May 4 — Changing Perspective

Yesterday, I picked sugar peas again. I worked all the rows twice, and then decided to look again in case I had missed any. I picked at least 30 percent more peas the third time, and wondered why I had missed so many. I had looked at the surface, and missed seeing the peas because they are the same color as the plant and easily blend with the leaves. A change of position, looking from another angle, gave me a different perspective and helped me to see those that were hidden.

Last fall, a similar thing happened when I gathered pecans. Charlie told me that hundreds of pecans had fallen under the trees, but when I first looked, I couldn't see them. I had to change my focus and look more closely. I first cleaned out the undergrowth around the tree. When I cleaned out the brush and old leaves and began to look closely, it was as though I had put on different glasses. I found hundreds of pecans.

The Lord is using these examples to show me something very applicable to what I am walking through. When I focus on the chemotherapy and its side effects, I miss the blessings—the fruit.

My perspectives of life, of crisis, of pain, and even of God have often been formed by

- experience,

- the influence of others,

- culture and tradition, and

- man's "religious" ideas, which don't always align
  with the Word of God.

Each of these influences can be a filter system, like cloudy or colored glasses, that keeps me from clearly seeing God's blessings. They can camouflage what God wants me to see. I am asking the Lord to show me what in my life hides His blessings, and to clean those things out of my life. He is faithful to show me what does not belong in my life and then to change me as I surrender those areas to Him.

In the past few months, God *is* changing my perspective. I pray daily for wisdom that allows me to see life through His eyes. I am allowing my understanding of life to be filtered through the Word of God. He has opened my spiritual eyes to see the blessings and the miracles. The new perspective makes each day a joy, even in the midst of pain. In fact, I am finding that the more difficult the situation seems to be, the deeper and more intently I look for His purposes and plans, and the larger and richer is the blessing.

So, I am picking peas . . . and ask forgiveness from those of you who thought everyone liked green peas. I promise that if you ever invite me to your house for dinner and you serve peas, I will be gracious and eat them. I will not hide them under the edge of the plate as I did when I was a kid!

🌿 GUEST

Mom, I've been reading Lamentations tonight — such a dark place for Jeremiah but still, amazingly, a place of hope. I'm so grateful that you have chosen to hope in the One who has never failed us, the One who never changes, though our circumstances do. . . .

God's loyal love could not have run out, his merciful love could not have dried up. They are created new every morning. How great is His faithfulness! I am sticking with God (I say it over and over). He is all I've got left.

> God proves to be good to the man who passionately waits, to the woman who diligently seeks. It's a good thing to quietly hope, quietly hope for help from God. It's a good thing . . . to stick it out through the hard times (Lamentations 3:25–27 MSG).

Love you and looking forward to Mom's Day. And we will NOT be having peas.

> When life is heavy and hard to take, go off by yourself. Enter the silence. Bow in prayer. Don't ask questions: Wait for hope to appear. Don't run from trouble. Take it full-face. The "worst" is never the worst. Why? Because the Master won't ever walk out and fail to return. If he works severely, he also works tenderly. His stockpiles of loyal love are immense" (Lamentations 3:28–33 MSG).

Christie

🌿 GUEST

How often do we miss God's blessings? I think I miss a bucketful. . . . Thank you for the reminder to look deeper, even into the things I did not like that day (doesn't have to be peas)! There they are, like pecans beneath the "undergrowth." Often it takes repentance to see beyond what I do not like and to appreciate it for the good God had packaged there. I do not want to miss the potential that God has planted in people and situations for His greater glory. Lord, help me to see with Your eyes. Meanwhile, sugar peas will never look the same to me after your stories. They will be sugar-pea reminders to look for God's blessings in everything.

I have been thinking about pain lately as it has come up in your journal. I remember something a pastor friend said, "There is no virtue in suffering." To that, I infer that, when suffering occurs, *we* determine the virtue that can come out of it. How do I respond through suffering in my life?

I am grateful that you have looked to a place beyond your pain and that you allow Jesus to direct your steps through it—so needed, not just in words but in deed. Thank you for being willing to be an example for tough encounters in life; what a difference it makes when Jesus is in the lead.

Grateful for our friendship and praying daily,

Dianna

🦋 GUEST

You have me looking at my circumstances from a different angle. Sure enough, you have more victories to celebrate when you find them tucked in the circumstances of life. I so appreciate our friendship and the wisdom you bring to my life.

Remember to let God carry you through the hardest spots and just rest against His breast. I had a dream last night of you in His arms with a big smile on your face. He really loves you and so do I.

Be blessed,
Joyce

Monday, May 5 — Experiencing Low WBC and Low Energy

I had a doctor's appointment this morning for blood tests. The doctor is monitoring me closely, and I feel well cared for!

Evidently, my body is not responding the way the doctor wants. Because I am not medically savvy, I don't know which numbers are supposed to be up and which are to be down. The doctor explained clearly, but I didn't write it down and I forgot. But when it comes to my WBC count and immune system, one number was supposed to be around 14 and was less than 1. The other number was supposed to be over 1000 and is less than 100. I do know that is not good. I met Carie for lunch afterward, and she explained some of it to me. Carie has helped me many times with her understanding of the medical terms and the implications of my condition.

Please pray that my WBC count begins to increase. I had a shot last Wednesday to boost the count, but it has not yet begun to do what my body needs. I started taking antibiotics again today to protect my immune system, and I go back for more blood tests on Thursday.

In the meantime, I am on my way to bed. Today, my energy has run out before the end of the day! I am so grateful that I have the freedom to do what my body tells me it needs.

Each day is different, but God is the same, and He does not change. He is steadfast. His faithfulness is always there, covering each situation, and He continues to provide the strength I need.

Wednesday, May 7 — Taking Rightful Control

I love living in the country. My office is a sunroom on the back of the house, overlooking the pastures. My study has many windows so I can see much of what happens outside. Yesterday morning, as I was sitting at my desk, a *huge* Texas longhorn (BEVO-style for you University of Texas people) walked past my window. She had escaped the pasture across the street and was wandering around, and she helped herself to a breakfast of my daisies. It made me smile.

I believe that one of the greatest benefits of my walking through the process of healing is that I am getting a crash course in how to minister to hurting people. I am not the standard for ministry or how to live a Godly life, but Jesus and the Holy Spirit — the Comforter — are the standard. I am learning about myself, as I have never walked through anything like this before. I am learning about God and how He views me and my situation. And, I am learning more about how to minister to others.

Today, I thought I would share some things the Lord has shown me that I believe will help me to minister more effectively to people in crisis.

Since I was diagnosed with cancer, I have lost control over some of the simple things of my life. Each of us has areas where we are not in control, but sometimes being in a crisis makes it much more obvious to us.

My body is still recovering from surgery, and I have places in my arm where I have no feeling and little strength. I have no hair, and I had no say as to whether it would fall out. The impact of chemotherapy is that I have no control over how my body reacts to the treatments. Some days, I have pain, nausea, no energy, and other reactions to the drugs.

In some areas of life, my control is only limited. I am now able to control some of my reactions to treatment through medication, which is an interesting challenge for someone who normally thinks twice before taking an aspirin. But I am grateful that I have medication to help.

I never thought about the "loss-of-control" issue until the Lord began to talk to me about it. I have thought that any control of my life is a bad thing that works against God being totally in control. But the Lord showed me that some "control" is rightfully mine, God-given, and I must be a good steward over that responsibility. To do that, I must set healthy boundaries for myself.

One of the most difficult things I have had to cope with is being asked about the details of my situation. When others let me set the agenda and tell only what I am comfortable sharing, I am blessed and relieved. I love the question, "Do you want to talk about it?" And I appreciate the freedom to say, "No." Much of the time, I am too tired to talk, which is the main reason for this website. I am grateful when people ask me how I am doing, but I am also glad when I don't have to give a lengthy answer. This will probably differ for each person. Some people like telling the details. Others want to share no details. By allowing the person in crisis the freedom to direct the conversation, you allow her to retain some of that rightful, God-given control.

Because we are each different, our needs and our reactions to each crisis will differ. One Sunday at church, a lady said, "I went through what you are going through, and I made it. One reason I made it was because I got so much attention. People were so kind to talk to me, to listen and do things for me. It was wonderful." I thanked her for sharing. And I had to laugh as I thanked the Lord for being so good to provide whatever we need. Her needs were almost the opposite of mine, as I have tried to avoid attention. I love that God knows each of us so completely and is able to meet our individual needs, no matter what those needs are.

I am asking the Lord to make me more sensitive to the needs of others. I want to minister to others according to what *they* need, not according to what *I* would need if I were in their situations. I don't want to project my feelings or needs on them. A number of people have said, "I know how you feel." (One was a man, and I wondered how he could relate to losing a breast.) Yet we are all different, and even when we walk through similar situations, we will have different perspectives and responses. For me, perhaps the most precious words I hear are "I am praying for you."

I have come to realize that not having experienced a situation does not keep me from ministering to a person any more than my going through a particular situation qualifies me. It all comes down to relying on the Holy Spirit to lead me with His love and compassion. I must not allow myself to be guided by my own fears, unresolved issues, unhealed hurts, or even my own experience.

If you are going through a crisis, I encourage you to decide what you want to share with other people. Be specific. Then decide in advance what you will graciously say when they ask you about something that you don't want to discuss. Then, and often the most difficult part, *do not give information that you do not want to share*. At times, I have shared things I did not want to share because I was afraid I would hurt people's feelings if I didn't answer their questions. (This people-pleasing thing is another issue that God is dealing with!) Then I struggled—not with them, but with myself—because I had violated what was best for me. You may be willing to share things with some people and not with others, and that's okay.

Also, if you are in a crisis, speak up for your wellbeing. If you have a need, express it. People will not know what you need if you don't tell them. For example, recently I have had to say to people, "Please do not hug me" or "Today is a no-hug day." We go to a very friendly church where people like to hug each other. But since I have started chemotherapy, much of the time I am in pain. At first it was difficult to ask people not to hug me, but after paying the painful price for silence several times, I decided to speak up. Also, with my immune system being low, the doctors have told me not to get close to people who are sick. I must speak up to protect myself.

The issue of protecting our boundaries applies to people in a variety of situations, not just those battling cancer. We must live our lives within healthy boundaries. God gives us authority and responsibility to determine our own boundaries, and calls us to respect others' boundaries. Violating those boundaries creates difficulty.

Ministry does not mean taking control of someone else's life or making decisions for them. Ministry does not mean telling them how to deal with their situation.

Ministry is encouragement. Ministry is pointing them to the Lord as He is the One who cares the most for them and who knows exactly how to deal with their problems.

And we are not to allow others to take control of our lives. That puts them in a place God never intended them to be. It is not always easy to take control of our lives and of the information of our situations. Other people don't always want to allow us that privilege. But it is important, even critical, for our own well-being and also for their well-being, for us to draw our boundaries and enforce them when necessary. It is not only unhealthy for us to allow others to come into our boundaries and take control, but it also unhealthy for them to be allowed to overstep their own boundaries. (If you want to read more about this, I highly recommend the book *Boundaries*.[19])

I am learning more about setting healthy boundaries and about taking the responsibility and control that is rightfully mine. I pray that the Lord will continue to teach me.

❧ GUEST

Your message today spoke to me very directly and touched me — thanks! Working day in and day out in health care, those of us in "the industry" tend to get a bit callous, not to the pain and suffering, but to the incredibly personal and invasive nature of health problems. I was recently caught off guard by a patient who was offended by my matter-of-fact discussion about her mammogram process, and it perhaps softened me to receive your message today with the right spirit. May the Lord bless you and yes, I will continue to pray for you — and all in the family.

Lee

ꙮ GUEST

Thank you immensely for such words of wisdom that are always timely. I want to read *Boundaries* again — actually, I need to read it carefully for the first time! All around me, mostly in me, I see the need for applying what you said in this journal entry. The message is encouraging and freeing. Working it out gets technical and seems uncertain, especially when someone like me has done a poor job of setting boundaries. But like you said, after I have paid the price a few times, living within my own boundaries proves so much better than hazarding to live outside of them. I find that I have to go back through my whole life to understand why I want to please others, why I hesitate to decline an invitation, and why I avoid confrontations. But really, understanding does not have to precede taking action that is good and right.

Pride is one reason why I hesitate to keep my own boundaries instead of accommodating someone else's — what would that person think of me? Insecurity is another reason. Ignorance is another. Fear is another. And compassion, unwisely expressed, is another. At least, those are thoughts that come to mind. Maturity helps. Personally, my hair, which I am more thankful for today than ever, is turning gray now, so I should be wiser with my age.

What you shared covers a lot of territory, and certainly the control issue has special significance to me. Personally, I tend to let the pendulum swing in the other direction, allowing myself to be controlled by someone else. So these are matters for prayer as I seek for wisdom and revelation — even plain common sense!

Thank you for the message. It is good to hear and prudent to apply.

Praying for more recruits among the "warrior cells,"

Dianna

ꙮ GUEST

Thank you for your wise words and for passing on to others what you are learning. I sometimes get caught up in the enormity of a given issue/crisis and I forget who I am and Whose I am. Then I begin to operate in the flesh and freeze up, not knowing what to say or do or how to act. In those situations, I frequently do nothing, fearing that I'll offend. On the outside, I appear to not care, but on the inside I want to do and say so many things. Thank you so much for helping me sort that out.

Thank you for graciously helping us help you. I continue to pray for you, my sister, and your family. I too sit at the computer with the tissues. I too am learning right along with you.

Much love,
Lissa

Friday, May 9—Having a Good Day

Yesterday, I had more blood tests. My WBC count had gone from 1 to 10, which is close to normal. YEA! The doctor was smiling! Thank you for the prayers. I have more energy today than I have had in a week so I'm trying to do a few things around the house. We also had an opportunity to minister to one of the nurses in the oncology office concerning some family matters. These trips to the doctor are always for more purposes than we think.

Thank you for all the encouragement. I have cried (so what else is new?) through your comments. I struggled with the last journal about whether to post it. I was so blessed to know that it had some value outside of my life.

Thursday, May 15—"Being" versus "Doing"

The Lord is working steadily during this time to change my perspective. This is not a new issue, but appears to be one that is taking a lifetime for me to understand.

I recently realized that most of my life I have been performance oriented, judging my personal worth on what I accomplish. I set goals for what I want to do, push myself to finish, and then rest . . . unless I have something else on my list that needs to be done immediately. At the end of the day, I normally decide if it has been a good day by looking back at what tasks I have accomplished. When I do not have visible completion to show what I have done, I feel like my day has not been successful. At present, I don't have enough energy to accomplish much. My goals are limited, and some days, all I can do is rest.

I know that in the Lord's eyes, our value is primarily based on our character rather than what we do. We are called human *beings*, not human *doings*. For me, the value of simply "being" is not an easy concept to grasp. It contradicts the values that I was taught as I grew up. I have always felt that I had to earn love and acceptance by doing good deeds. But the Lord keeps bringing me back to face this issue. He faithfully demonstrates His principles to me in graphic and sometimes humorous ways.

Charlie brought me an unexpected Mother's Day gift—a puppy. Unbeknownst to me, he had seen puppies at a neighbor's house. Last Friday, we were coming home from town and the owner was in the yard with all the puppies. We stopped to take a closer look. When we left, we took one home with us.

We have considered getting a dog for years, but every time I thought about the responsibility, I concluded it was not at the top of my list. Contrary to my human reasoning, we had peace that now is the right time, and we have adopted "Wasco." I won't bore you with the detailed story behind that, other than to say he is named for a town in California that we drove through 18 years ago. We decided if we ever had a dog, we would name him after that small friendly town. So, Wasco it is.

The other day, I went outside to work and Wasco went with me. When I was sitting on the ground in the garden, he was in my lap. When I was on my knees, he was sitting on the backs of my legs. He was next to me the entire time, though it was hot and he was panting. This puppy doesn't want Charlie or me to go anywhere without him. He sits at our feet if we won't let him sit in our laps. He is presently in my lap, and I am dealing with two paws on the computer keyboard and his teeth on the mouse.

So, what do we do? When he wants to go outside and play, we drop everything and go run with him. When he cries at 5 a.m., and it sounds like "I need to go," we get up and take him outside and then spend time playing with him. We make sure he has all that he needs. But he wants *to be with us* more than anything. He is a puppy and does things we don't especially like, but we are training him. And we love him and especially enjoy that he wants to be with us. This is so different from our cats that are very independent and self-sufficient.

The Lord began speaking to me in the garden about the puppy. He said, "This is my heart. I, too, love it when you stay close to me, even when it is hot and you are tired. When you desire Me and simply enjoy My presence, will I not give you everything you need?"

Being with the Lord is what He wants. I can't earn His love, His favor, His promises, or His blessing. My heavenly Father simply gives them to me, His child. He wants to take care of me.

I desire more than anything to stay close to Him. I feel the Lord near when I hurt. And I feel Him near when I am happy and healthy. I cannot see God with my physical eyes, but I do see evidence of His presence. I *know* He is with me. That is not just mental knowing or "blind faith." I hear His voice. I feel His peace inside. His presence is real, and the love and joy He gives is amazing and comforting. All I have to do is draw near to Him (James 4:8a NASB). I am thankful for His love and that He does not turn away when we are hurting or needy or failing or not accomplishing all we want. And He does not remove His presence when we are sick.

Tomorrow, I have another heart scan and next Tuesday I have the third round of chemotherapy, and the process begins again. In the midst of all the challenges, I continue to sing of His faithfulness and "It is well with my soul!".[20]

GUEST

Good morning, friend! . . . Oh, how the Lord loves you . . . speaks your name across the universe and into the hearts of many . . . placing your face before Himself and the bride . . . what a God we belong to . . . and this is His conversation this morning:

> One generation shall praise Your works to another, and shall declare Your mighty acts. On the glorious splendor of Your majesty and on Your wonderful works, I will meditate. Men shall speak of the power of Your awesome acts, and I will tell of Your greatness. They shall eagerly utter the memory of Your abundant goodness and will shout joyfully of Your righteousness (Psalm 145:4–7 NASB).

I'm shouting . . .
CJ

GUEST

Thanks so much for logging your thoughts and what God is continuing to do in your life!

God recently showed me that my primary love language is quality time. What I was missing in this revelation was that God wants me to engage my love language of quality time with *Him*! This is sort of new, but also very natural, to me. Like you stated in your journal, my past has been performance driven. . . . I feel I have to *show* God that I love Him by doing, and if I don't *do*, then I feel I don't love Him as much as I should.

Now, I'm endeavoring to first *be* with God and then *do* with God . . . the first step kills the performance stuff, and the second step allows the Love that I gain from Him to be shared with others. It's similar to the fact that when God created the first day (Genesis 1:5), it was evening (a time of resting) and then morning (a time of doing). To me, it seems that morning should come first, . . . but that's not God's design. I'm so glad we have a loving Father who is patient in teaching us *His* ways!

Keep resting in Him!
Lana

GUEST

Good morning. I hope you are using your "strong" days to relax and to enjoy that puppy! I can't wait to meet him.

The children and I continue to study how God favors those who seek Him. Today's lesson was about Hezekiah the Israelite king. When the king of Assyria came against the Israelites, Hezekiah, who was righteous, called on God, and the Angel of the Lord destroyed the enemy (2 Chronicles 32).

So, as your website encourages friends and family to call upon the Lord, may He continue to multiply your "warrior cells" and may His angel destroy the enemy cells in your body!

Love you!
Carie

Monday, May 19 — Preparing for Treatment 3

If all goes well with tests tomorrow, around noon I will have chemotherapy treatment 3. The treatment should take 3–4 hours. I am not fearful, for which I am very thankful. I am keeping my mind focused on the Lord and the people around me, rather than on what is happening to my body.

In the past, the day of the treatment was not difficult. If this one is like the last two, I will be tired when it is over, but I will not immediately have pain. I have not been nauseated either. I am grateful and consider my lack of side effects to be a *huge* answer to prayers.

The day after chemotherapy is usually a good day also. I begin to experience the impact of the chemicals on my body within 36–48 hours. At least now, I have an idea of what to expect. In the past, the more difficult side effects began on Wednesday night or Thursday morning and lasted for about 10 days. I have medication to control some of the pain.

Today, I am trying to get the house in order so that my schedule in the coming week is easier. In the past five days, I have had no energy, so I am working a little and then resting. We even stayed home from church yesterday, as I didn't have the energy to get showered and dressed. Today is a beautiful day and after resting yesterday, I have been able to accomplish some necessary chores. Charlie mowed the yard after he got the lawn mower, weed eater, and vacuum cleaner running. He had a full morning of repairing broken tools, which is never fun. I often tease him, telling him he can fix anything but me!

At of the end of this day, I will be one-third of the way through chemotherapy, and after the next three weeks, I will be one-half of the way through. It seems like months since I began treatment, but I continue to try to learn from every experience and challenge, and am thankful for the healing process that is taking place.

Friday, May 23—Learning the Meaning of "Rest"

Tuesday, I had the third chemotherapy treatment. My WBC count was up and my heart-strength numbers have increased. In the past three days, I have slept much. The fatigue is increasing, so I am learning how to take naps, which is not so difficult when my body stops going.

The bigger challenge is how to balance activity and rest. I have some new insights to what it means to "rest." In the past, my idea of "resting" has been to do something that doesn't take as much energy, such as to read or watch an old movie while sewing or working on a craft. Or sometimes "rest" has meant to completely crash from exhaustion or burn out.

When Charlie was on active duty, his vacation days often meant that he didn't go into the office until 9 a.m., he worked a short day, or he wore civilian clothes rather than his uniform when he went to the office. When we lived in Hawaii, our concept of a day of "rest" was to pack a large picnic lunch, bath towels, bathing suits, and lawn chairs and head to the beach. We would drive across the island to spend the day, play, pack up, drive home, do laundry, and put everything away, and often go to bed exhausted from a full day of fun. When Charlie and I go on a vacation, it is more likely a trip like when we went to Israel. We awoke at 6 a.m., were on a bus at 8 a.m., toured all day, returned to the hotel for dinner, and then had a study session from 7–9 p.m. We often think of rest as a change of pace and place. In the busy world we live in, rest often has different and relative meanings.

My idea of rest is shifting. With my energy being limited, rest sometimes means *no* activity rather than *less* activity! This is a new concept and discipline for me, yet, I am beginning to see how essential rest is to my entire life and not just to the healing process from chemotherapy. I believe it will be important to my quality of life in the future.

For Mother's Day, Carie gave me a gift that I have wanted for years: a copy of the 1828 Noah Webster Dictionary. It is amazing how Webster used Scriptures in his definitions. He defines "rest" as

> To cease from action or motion of any kind; rest from mental exertion; rest of body or mind. A body is at rest when it ceases to move; the mind is at rest when it ceases to be disturbed or agitated; the sea is never at rest. Hence, quiet, repose, a state free from motion or disturbance; a state of reconciliation to God. To stop work, applicable to anybody or being, and to any kind of motion. To cease from labor, work or performance. . . . God rested on the 7th day from all his work which he has made (Genesis 2). So the people rested on the 7th day (Exodus 16). To be quiet or still; to be undisturbed. To be quiet or tranquil, as the mind; not to be agitated by fear, anxiety or other passion.[21]

This definition defines a quality of rest as well as a state of rest — "at peace" and unlike the sea. Rest is a state of mind as well as a discipline for the body. I see why the writer of Hebrews indicates that it takes faith to enter into rest (Hebrews 3:18–4:3). It is more than sleep or inactivity. Rest is an attitude of confidence in the Lord that involves faith and hope, trusting (resting in) His care and giving thanks for all God is doing and is going to do. That becomes very real in the midst of pain or uncertainty.

In our busy society, we are bombarded with constant noise that often makes rest illusive. However, at this unique time of my life, when so many things — activities, habits, priorities, as well as preconceived ideas and standards — are having to be laid down, I am truly finding some valuable keys to life. True rest is one of those keys. It is not rest from exhaustion but is rest in the midst of my situation, in the midst of the storm.

Our culture is full of man-made noises. When I am in a store, office, or restaurant where there is loud music or a television, it drains my energy. One of the most important elements of rest has become the "quiet." Sometimes that is silence; sometimes that is listening to the birds sing, the chorus of frogs croaking, or the creek running. Those sounds of nature bring energy to my body.

Isaiah 30:15 (NKJV) says at the beginning of the verse, "In returning and rest you shall be saved; In quietness and confidence shall be your strength." In the quiet, I gain strength, whereas when I am in noisy places, I lose strength. When all is quiet, I find it much easier to hear God's still small voice (1 Kings 19:12), sense His presence, and feel His strength pouring into me.

A friend told us that our home in the country was a hidden place of refuge. That is very true. The quiet of our home, with all the sounds of nature, provides a safe, restful and healing place for me.

Thank you for the continued prayers. This journey is a "long stretch," and I know that staying the course and supporting over the long haul can be exhausting. I can't tell you how much I appreciate your continued love and encouragement.

❧ GUEST

Please know that even as you rest, you accomplish so much: you testify to truth to many, you teach your children and grandchildren, and you glorify the Kingdom. Your journal entry on rest was particularly potent — and I love seeing you grow (and continue to learn from you) and flourish.

You looked terrific today—may I say it again? And I'm so proud of your attitude of dignity, even when you are weary.

Love,
Carie

✤ GUEST

I have been amazed and encouraged by the beauty of your testimony in the midst of struggles. I thank God for your witness.

I, too, have had to learn about rest. Several years ago, I went through a time of depression and the Lord's word to me was "Rest." I received His message from every direction and knew it was from Him. I received spiritual help from my pastor, among others, and after the first week, I went back to him and said, "This week I have rested. Now what?" He just laughed at me and said, "Keep resting." Here I am four years later and still learning what a gracious, tender word that is—to rest. The Webster's definition was rich; thank you for passing that along. When my need was great, God supplied me with help and healing from many sources, and now I pray that He will continue to do the same for you. You and Charlie and the family are in my prayers.

With fond thoughts of our friendship,

Jan

✤ GUEST

Thank you for inspiring us to truly rest. That's one thing I actually enjoyed and embraced last year as I went through cancer treatment. I have to admit it was hard to get back into all the daily duties of a mom. I sometimes long for those days when I had a good excuse to just stop whatever I was doing and go sit or lie down without being disturbed.

I'm so glad to hear that your blood counts and heart numbers are stable and everything is on track.

Praying for you! Enjoy your rest.

Susan

"He who dwells in the shelter of the Most High will rest in the shadow of the Almighty" (Psalm 91:1).

Wednesday, May 28 — Cleaving in Sickness and in Health

Today, Charlie and I are celebrating our 41st wedding anniversary. I am filled with gratitude and excitement as I look back and see all God has done in us through the past four decades. We were not the same people 41 years ago that we are today. Marriage is hard work, and we have both changed, but it has certainly been worth it.

I remember walking down the aisle to become the wife of that nice-looking, young lieutenant whom I barely knew. He was commissioned into the Air Force the day before we were married. That was really great, as he has never forgotten our anniversary.

We did not know each other very long before we married, and we both quickly came to the realization that we did not especially like each other. Thus, our lives together began!

Our marriage is an amazing testimony of God's power and faithfulness, plus the dedication of one man to God. It was through my faithful husband, his commitment to the Lord, his constant demonstration of grace, and his prayers that I came to know the Lord.

I have looked back and laughed many times at something Charlie said shortly after we got married, "Everything that is mine is mine and everything that is yours is mine." Back then, I thought that was a "possession thing" — a proclamation of his right of ownership. I did not have a bank account, money of my own, a car in my name. Even my name was changed to his. Yet, through the years, as we lived our lives together, I came to understand that his statement represented his willingness to take responsibility for leading our family and taking care of me and our children.

In the past five months, those words have taken on a much deeper meaning — that everything that is mine is also his. He has taken this journey as something *we* are walking through rather than something *I* am walking through. He has not been an observer but a participant. Sometimes, I even think he feels my pain as much as I do.

During these months, Charlie has taken on much added responsibility. He has done many practical things such as cook meals, wash dishes, do laundry, and clean house. He has gone to numerous doctor's appointments, held my hand when I got my hair all cut off, laughed with me, allowed me to cry and even cried with me on occasion, held me, encouraged me, and spent countless hours simply listening. And then to look at this bald woman and tell her she looks beautiful — that is a priceless treasure! I have truly come to appreciate and understand the preciousness of "for better, for worse, in sickness and in health, 'til death do us part" and even the price one pays to live that commitment.

One of the greatest things Charlie's life has taught me is that marriage is not a 50–50 deal. His idea of marriage has always been that marriage is 100–100. Both of us have to be willing to give 100%, and sometimes we have to do that when the other person is not willing or able to give anything at all. That is a beautiful picture, not only of the Lord, but also of servanthood. Charlie has lived that principle throughout our marriage and even more during the past five months.

Today, I am filled with gratitude for the many gifts of grace and sacrificial love that I have received but that I do not deserve, especially the gift of my husband.

Thank you to all of you who have prayed specifically for him as he continues to give, to serve, and to take care of me.

❧ GUEST

Dear Sweetheart,

Happy Anniversary! Forty-one years ago today our Heavenly Father gave me my greatest earthly gifts: your love and the privilege of sharing life with you. Following the privilege of serving the Lord, our marriage has been and continues to be the second most important source of joy and purpose in my life. Thank you for your faithfulness, encouragement, and stamina and a daily exemplary life that has brought hope, purpose, and vision to me and thousands of people around the world.

Anniversaries bring back memories, and we have shared so many together. Every one of them is special:

- Celebrating our anniversary in Holland on the way home from teaching in the Baikal Bible School in Siberia.

- Praying together at Caesarea Philippi.

- Being serenaded by a cuckoo bird on our way to Sunday church in Seoul, Korea.

- Watching the sun set on Waikiki Beach.

- Talking on the MARS shortwave military radio between you in Dallas and me in Southeast Asia, having to say "over" each time we wanted to hear each other.

Or, some other "big-ees" like stringing barbed-wire fences or shopping at Half Price Books. And this year, sharing Wasco with the world via CaringBridge.org. Whatever the "event," what made it most special was enjoying it together.

Over the course of our marriage, you have often told people that at the wedding altar, I said to you, "Whatever I have is mine and whatever you have is also mine." I honestly don't remember saying that, although it's not a bad philosophy, and time often proves that your memory of such important matters is better than mine.

But this year, we are sharing something unlike any past anniversaries. And what you "have" truly is mine because we are passing along the journey of this season together, knowing that God is our Victor and Healer and that He will rule and reign to the revelation of His glory in this matter of your health and your complete healing.

Thank you again for your exemplary encouragement, affirmed and honored by so many who read what you share here, and who go about life with a clearer understanding of *who* they are because of *Whose* they are and the price He paid for their salvation.

I love you more than even 41 years of marriage can say. I am *very proud* of you and blessed to know you are my best friend.

Never forget the character of God: more than taking you *from* something, He takes you *to* something, and He always saves the best for last. We are on a journey to prepare us for a new and more powerful Kingdom calling. Life together has been wonderful, and the best part, in the years ahead and then in eternity, is yet to come.

Your devoted husband,
Charlie

❧ GUEST

Happy 41st Anniversary! I've thought of y'all so much today and have to thank God for your faithfulness to each other and to your commitment. Thank you for that legacy for your children and grandchildren and that example for others! We claim that for generations to come.

Much love to both of you today! I'm so proud of you!

Carie

❧ GUEST

Who knew that a young lieutenant and his unsaved bride would have changed the world 41 years later? Who knew that the Book of Life would have to add pages because of the impact you two have made for the Kingdom? It's a privilege to have watched you and Daddy, with such determination, grow together through changes and seasons and always end up loving each other more because of it.

Happy Celebrating!
Christie

❧ GUEST

Thank you for sharing so transparently about your marriage, your growth, the bridegroom and the bride becoming one—what a beautiful picture. You and Charlie offer such inspiration! May your latter years together keep on getting better!

Our society does not encourage doing what you two did—persevering even when life is not fun. Our society misses the fruit of patient endurance, denying yourself and really loving someone else beside yourself! What unique hope we have as Christians that we can do all things through Christ, that our God is the God of hope and that love never fails. May the grace of our Lord continue to mark your lives.

Love always,
Dianna

Friday, May 30 — Giving the Gift of Time

For someone in a crisis, time can either be a friend or an enemy. With cancer, the process of treatment and healing takes time, but I also talk to many patients who are fearful that in time the cancer will reappear in their bodies.

I have heard the statements, "Time is on my side" and "Time heals all wounds." I am not sure that those are absolute truths, though some things do take time. The process to heal or to change does not always happen immediately. It may not always be the time itself that heals, but time does give us the opportunity to deal with issues.

I read a friend's article on CaringBridge about the importance of time for her baby who needs a heart transplant and needs to heal from a long-term infection. She mentioned that new medical discoveries are being made very quickly, and things are possible today that could not be done even 6–12 months ago. I think of a friend who may not have much time to live, according to doctor's predictions. We must each face the future, not knowing how much time we have left on this earth.

My experience of time is interesting. Some days seem to go by far too quickly while others seem to go by in slow motion. Charlie recently reminded me that though each of us is created different with unique abilities, talents, and gifts, we are each equally given the same 24 hours a day. The question is not, "How much time do I have?" but "What will I do with the time I do have?"

Some people simply allow time to pass. For others, time becomes an investment and is that which allows them to achieve goals.

I want to take an active and aggressive approach to my future and to using the gift of time that God has given to me. That decision is being made on a daily basis, as I use each minute, each hour wisely. It comes down to the choices I make, as those choices determine what the results will be.

God has much to say about the subject of "time." He created the lights to divide day from night and be signs for seasons, days, and years (Genesis

1:14–19.) Time is contained *within* the eternal unlimited God. He sees the beginning and the end at the same time. He is not impacted, controlled, or hindered by time, distance, or any of the other limitations that confine man. Yet, He created time and gave it to us as a gift.

So often, this word appears in the Scriptures as "the appointed time" or "in due time," which often refer to seed planting or harvest, seasons of time, or childbirth. Scriptures also state "in the fullness of time" and usually precede prophecy given or prophecy fulfilled. In the Psalms, a number of times David writes, "in time of trouble" and then follows with testimony of God's loving deliverance for His people.

One of my favorite Scriptures is in the book of Esther when Mordecai is encouraging Queen Esther to risk her life and speak to the King in order to save the Jewish nation:

> For if you keep silent at this time, relief and deliverance will rise for the Jews from another place, but you and your father's house will perish. And who knows whether you have not come to the kingdom *for such a time as this*? (Esther 4:14 ESV, emphasis added).

This Scripture refers to her destiny, the reason why God chose her to become the Queen and perhaps why she was born. Esther did approach the King, and the Jewish race was saved because of her obedience. As with Esther, I want to be obedient and fulfill the destiny God has for my life.

Another familiar passage is when King Solomon writes

> To everything there is a season, and a time to every purpose under the heavens: a time to be born, and a time to die; a time to plant, and a time to pluck up that which is planted . . . a time to weep, and a time to laugh . . . a time to keep silence, and a time to speak; a time to love, and a time to hate; a time of war, and a time of peace (Ecclesiastes 3:1–2, 4a, 7a–8 Darby).

He follows that with another of my favorite Scriptures, "(God) has made everything beautiful in its time. He has also set eternity in the hearts of men . . ." (Ecclesiastes 3:11a–b).

I want to be aware of and ready for the seasons of life and to walk through each gracefully. Rather than become discouraged with my limitations, I want to rejoice in the things I *can* do and pursue doing all that is within my capabilities.

As a gift from God, time can be a valuable resource, especially if we use it according to His guidance. One morning recently, Charlie prayed a prayer that has become a daily prayer for me:

> Lord, at the end of this day, may we not measure our
> success by our accomplishments, but by our obedience
> to do your will.

Then, we wait patiently for Him to make *all* things beautiful, just as He has promised. "And we know that God causes all things to work together for good to those who love God, to those who are called according to *His* purpose" (Roman 8:28 NASB). For His children, nothing can defeat us when we surrender to His loving and powerful hand.

Many people have spent time through the years praying for Charlie and me, our marriage, our ministry, and our family. The testimony of our lives would not be the same had those people not invested the gift of prayer. Many have also taken time to pray for my health during the past five months. Some of those people don't even know me, but they have invested their time to seek the Father's best for my life. What a gift!

This week, I was given a "prayer blanket" from people at the First Methodist Church in our town. One lady made the blanket, and at church last Sunday, many people came forward and tied knots in the fringe of the blanket as they prayed for me. Charlie and I are not members of that church and many of them do not know us, but they know the power of prayer and were willing to pray on my behalf.

A number of people have prepared food for us and driven long distances to deliver the meal. Others have written encouraging cards, notes, and emails. Many of you are doing these kinds of things for dozens of people. All of that is an investment of your limited resource of time into something that has eternal value and that pleases God.

As I think of all of you who have spent time ministering to me, I see it as a visual demonstration of your love for Christ and for the members of His body. Ahhhh . . . that the world would see that love and know that Jesus came!

Sunday, June 1 — Catching a Glimpse of Normal Life

Thank you for your prayers. God is hearing and answering. I have felt better during the last week than I have since I began chemotherapy. This round has been very different. I have had very few side effects and only about 48 hours of pain, which was mild!

When I went in for a blood test last Tuesday, my WBC count was high enough that, for the first time, I didn't have to take antibiotics. When I went back on Friday, my WBC count was normal! I have had more energy than I have had in months and have led almost a "normal" life for the past week. I have even been able to work outside in the flowerbeds and the garden early in the mornings and a few times after dinner. I am rejoicing.

The nurse told me it was nice for me to have a couple of "good days." I think she was trying to tell me that it might not be typical, but I know much of this is because of prayer. Thank you! Just wanted to share the good report!

❧ GUEST

You go, girl!! How wonderful that you are doing so well. Now you can join me in encouraging other women facing this that chemo is *do-able*—not enjoyable by any means, but do-able. I'll bet that mountain doesn't seem quite as big as it did a few months ago, does it? I'll pray for more of these good days throughout your treatment.

Love,
Susan

❧ GUEST

To God be the glory, and Mom, you are too modest to say so, but you look *beautiful*! As Susan said, you are showing others that chemo is do-able, but you are doing so much more. You continue to worship and apply your strength to pointing to God, whether you are at the clinic, in nuclear medicine, or in a store shopping.

May God continue to defy the odds with you.

(And thanks to all of those precious people who have provided meals, sent beautiful flowers, and posted on this website. Your encouragement is so precious to our family!)

Carie

I listened yesterday to a sermon by Louie Giglio. He shared that when one endures suffering and difficulties, the Lord gives you a megaphone to shout to all, "I trust God and nothing separates me from His love." So, I thank our Lord for your megaphone so you can shout "God is good all the time," and know we are hearing you loud and clear.

Much love,
Vicky

Tuesday, June 10 — Giving Honor and Grace

I am grateful that I know I am going *through* this situation; there is an end. The Lord spoke to me at the beginning, that *this was not unto death*. However, many of the people I meet do not have that assurance. They only know that they are in the middle of a situation, and they do not know the outcome. Many are fearful. This week, I prayed with a man in the office who has chemotherapy the same days I do and has had 28 treatments. I also talked to a lady on experimental drugs who was told she would die six years ago. It is a privilege when I get to encourage them, and especially when I get to pray for them.

I remember times when I would meet someone in a difficult situation, and I would not know what to say, so I would say nothing. Now, I approach those people to listen or to say something kind. God has truly given me compassion and increased my boldness.

Sunday morning, we sang a new chorus at church and the words were simple yet struck a chord in my heart, "Glorify Your name above all names".[22] Recently, the phrase "name above all names" has been especially powerful to me. To know that the name of Jesus is more powerful than the name of cancer, fear, depression, discouragement, hopelessness, intimidation, and even death brings great peace to my heart.

What does it mean that His name is "above" other names? His character and nature, the essence of who He is, is reflected in His name. He is sovereign God, Ruler of heaven and earth. We do not use the name of Jesus like a good-luck charm, but we put our trust in His character, His Word, and all He has done for us.

I asked the Lord to show me how to glorify His name, not just in words but also in a practical way in my present situation and in the future. When we got home from church, I looked up the definition of "to glorify" and found that it has the same meaning as "to honor," which means "to prize, to not take lightly, to esteem, to give weight to, to ascribe worth," and especially "to highly value".[23]

Of course, God — our Creator, Savior, Giver of Life — should receive honor and glory. I find that I can easily glorify and honor Him, especially with my words and songs, because He truly is worthy. But I also want to honor Him with my thoughts, attitudes, and actions and in the practical areas of life. If I have no action to go with my words, my words are empty.

God has reminded me of the simple truth that each person whom He created is worthy of honor because each person is made in His image. Often I have honored people because of what they did. Now I see that difficult, unjust, and seemingly undeserving people also need honor and love. *They may have no idea that God thinks they are valuable.* Giving them what they have not earned or deserved is giving grace. God poured out His grace on us, and we are to pour out grace on others.

Giving honor is like giving love as it depends on the person giving it, rather than the person receiving it. When we honor people, we are demonstrating God's character, His love, and His grace. And as we honor others, we are honoring Him. He loved us enough to die for us while we were still sinners (Romans 5:8); we are to go and share that same life with others, even those walking in sin.

We can easily put value on our own lives, but the test is when we put that same value on the lives of others, no matter who they are. The Lord wants us to look at every person with His eyes, and then affirm their value, worth, and potential.

This truth should be obvious to me. Yet, the Holy Spirit is bringing this truth to my attention as I face this new situation. God's Word tells us to love every person, including our enemies. And He says that when we do something kind to the "least of these," we are doing it to Him (Matthew 25:40). I have known this for years, but I find that it is easier to talk about treating every person with love and honor than it is to put that into action.

And I cannot do this on my own. Love for all people comes only with God's help and through the work of His Spirit. It is easier for me to go into the hospital, a restaurant, or a shopping center and keep to myself, ignoring others. When I am with someone I do not agree with or do not like, I can focus on myself and what I need rather than considering the other person's needs. However, through my present situation, I am becoming aware that everywhere people are in need. My daily prayer has become that I reach beyond myself and honor every person I meet, thus glorifying and honoring God with my actions.

Last week, the oncologist said everything is going well with me physically, and he scheduled my next treatment for tomorrow. As of today, I am halfway through the treatment.

God is answering your prayers in abundance. I am grateful for all the opportunities I am having, opportunities to change, to learn, to touch lives, to see life with a different perspective. I pray that will continue. Also, in the past few weeks, I have felt good physically, and I am grateful. Now, I face the next treatment trusting that He will provide all I need as He has in the past weeks.

❧ GUEST

This journal entry again has so much worth sharing with the body of Christ. "Lord, forgive us for our prejudices that have led to treating one another differently based on how we look, sit, walk, or stand. Help us . . . deliver us from ourselves." Thank you again, Suzanne. . . . May your words find the eyes, ears, and minds of those who need encouragement. . . .

Many times I have felt overwhelmed by a person obviously in great need and have not known what to say or do, yet your testimony makes giving an encouraging response so natural and simple. Just . . . letting the Lord fill my mouth (if I believe that I should say or do something but don't know what) could make an eternal difference in someone's life. . . .

Love and prayers,
Dianna

Friday, June 13 — Preparing for the Future

Thank you for the continued precious gift of your prayers. I had chemo treatment 4 on Wednesday. The treatment was not too difficult, but I had a long day, as we attended church Wednesday evening and a meeting afterwards.

Yesterday, Charlie drove me to Frisco to get a WBC booster shot. It took three hours to get there and home for a 30-second shot. I slept most of the rest of the day. I had some nausea, but it is gone now.

I was awake for several hours during the night. As I spent that time praying, some interesting thoughts came to mind. One is how it seems that we more easily turn to the Lord when we face a crisis.

Last year was an easy year, without crisis, yet the Lord did much work in my life. That work prepared and strengthened me for my present situation. He knew what was ahead when I did not know.

We must spend time with Him when things are going smoothly. My tendency has often been to coast in my relationship with the Lord when things are going well. When I do, I can miss valuable things He wants to do in and through me.

Even in the military, the troops practice for war during times of peace. When war comes, they have no time to prepare. They must prepare beforehand.

A farmer uses the winter to work on his equipment. If he waits until planting or harvest time to get his equipment in shape, he will not be ready at the proper time. If Charlie waits until spring when the grass is high before he gets the mowers running, the job is much more difficult than if he spends time during the fall and winter preparing for the spring.

We never know what is ahead, but God does, and He is faithful to prepare us when we cooperate with Him and regularly seek Him.

Another interesting thing that came to mind is that of walking in the Spirit, as Paul talks about in Romans 8. Difficult circumstances can easily pull us down like gravity, but when we walk in the Spirit, circumstances do not control us, and we can rise above them.

Last night, despite nausea and pain, I retreated into the refuge of the Lord. As I did, I was surrounded with His presence. Not only was I filled with amazing peace and my stomach calmed, but He filled me with such joy that I found myself, even in the dark, smiling and laughing. God's presence is amazing. When we focus on Him rather than on ourselves, He *becomes* what we need. In His presence there is peace, joy, strength, and healing. He gives Himself to us freely. How amazing is God's love for us.

So, the journey continues. This is a process, not just an event. Your faithful encouragement and prayers are a priceless gift to me that I will never be able to repay. I pray the Lord will richly reward each of you for your impact on my life. You will never know how much you mean to me!

Monday, June 16 — Seeing God's Grace for Every Situation

Today is a good day. The weekend was painful — definitely "no hug" days. I don't know if the pain was from the chemotherapy or the WBC booster shot. However, this morning when I woke up, much of the pain had subsided. I am getting ready to take a nap at 11 a.m., as exhaustion and other side effects have set it. None are overwhelming but just need attending. During my life, I have often ignored my body and would insist that it simply submit to the situation. Recently, however, I am listening to what my body needs and am learning to take care of it. So, today is a day of rest and taking care of my "shell!"

A friend recently told Charlie that he didn't know what to say to me and that he could not go through cancer the way I am because I seem so strong. First, encouragement is a blessing, and knowing people are standing with me is a gift. Second, I feel anything but strong. I am learning to press into the Lord more for *His* strength, which is different from my own. My strength runs out quickly; His lasts forever. Mine is outward and physical; His is inside. As Christians, we are to lean on and trust Him in whatever situations we walk through. I am so grateful for His truth that says, "My grace is sufficient for you, for My strength is made perfect in weakness" (2 Corinthians 12:9 NKJV). I truly qualify, as I am weak in so many ways, and I recognize my weakness more each day. Grace is the divine ability that allows us to do what God has called us to do, even through difficult situations. I daily pray for His strength to be made perfect in me and for His grace to sustain and enable me.

This morning, I talked to a mother whose son is an alcoholic, and I thought, "I could not go through that." I thought of a friend recently widowed and wondered how she can handle that situation. Each of us, however, has grace for whatever we face. The enemy of our souls will send anything he can to steal, kill, and destroy our lives and our families (John 10:10), as his plan is for us to turn away from God. But when we trust God, He overcomes all the plots and schemes of the enemy. I have the grace to walk through the situations of my own life; you have grace to walk through the challenges in yours. Honestly, when I look at what other people have to face, my challenges often look easy, but only because God's grace is at work in my life. Trusting Him, therefore, is possible in the midst of my journey.

I remember a conversation from years ago when my children were small. My sister and I were talking about our lives. She said, "I don't see how you stand it!" She was referring to my life as a military wife and the way we moved (19 times in 26 years) — leaving friends, making new ones, establishing a new home every few years, and facing the other challenges that come with frequent moves. For her, that was more than she could handle, but for me, life was exciting, and I eagerly anticipated what was ahead. Ironically, I had been thinking the same thing about her life because she had lived for years in one place and was not expecting to move for many years. Plus, she had to "spring clean" and I didn't. I simply moved when the house got dirty!

I have only *my* life to live and I am leaning on Him and His grace to walk in victory. God is sufficient for all I must face. He is the answer for each of us. No situation is too big for Him, if we will only trust Him and ask Him to be God over the situations of our lives.

Today, He is Lord over weariness and over the healing process, and I have joy in simply being alive. Today, may He be Lord over every challenge you are facing and may you find Him faithful to pour out His grace on your life. He is willing and able.

ꙮ GUEST

Dear Sweetheart,

Your writing on the grace of God reminded me again of one of my all-time favorite songs, "He Giveth More Grace," by Annie Johnson Flint. It's one I sing often when I'm outside working, and especially as I walk with you through the journey of this season of your life.

> He giveth more grace when the burdens grow greater,
> He sendeth more strength when the labors increase,
> To added affliction He addeth His mercy,
> To multiplied trials, His multiplied peace.
>
> When we have exhausted our store of endurance,
> When our strength has failed ere the day is half-done,
> When we reach the end of our hoarded resources,
> Our Father's full giving is only begun.

His love has no limit, His grace has no measure,
His power has no boundary known unto men;
For out of His infinite riches in Jesus,
He giveth and giveth and giveth again.[24]

I love you Sweetheart!
Charlie

"For of His fullness we have all received, and grace upon grace"
(John 1:16 NASB).

❧ GUEST

I was thinking about you this afternoon and recalled this Scripture:
"I consider that our present sufferings are not worth comparing
with the glory that will be revealed in us" (Romans 8:18).

Someday, God will ask each of us how we each faced the trials He
allowed in our lives. (He allowed them but did not necessarily
cause them.) We will each have to answer for our behavior, and as
you answer for how you faced this struggle, God will be
glorified — and that glory will be exponentially greater than the
pain and suffering you faced in your circumstances.

May your "warrior cells" multiply today, and may you rest in the
fact that He is "growing glory" in you through even this. And may
He bless you *now* on earth for your faithfulness to direct others'
eyes to Him as the source of your strength and joy.

Love,
Carie

Wednesday, June 18 — Knowing God Cares for Us

Yesterday, I had to go to the hospital for blood tests, which was more
exciting than I had anticipated. I arrived at the hospital in a major
downpour with winds of up to 70 mph. I believed it wise that I not get
soaked walking through the storm, so I sat in the car for thirty minutes.
The rain did not slacken, so I decided to pick up lunch through the drive-
thru at Chick-Fil-A and then return to the hospital. As a result, it took from

10:45 a.m. to 3:30 p.m. to go to the hospital, have my blood drawn, and return home!

The test showed that my WBC count, which should be 10–14, was 0.9 and the "good cells" were only at 0.3. I have come to appreciate WBCs and understand the impact they have on my body and on how I feel. So, today I am resting. I am praying that those warrior cells multiply and do their work. The doctor put me on antibiotics to guard from infection until the cells begin to multiply. The nurse said the WBC booster shot should "kick in," which is an accurate description of how it feels. However, the shot has not done its "kicking in" yet, so I pray that will begin soon. I return on Friday for more blood tests.

A friend made a statement that has really ministered to me today — that God does not just care *about* His children, which indicates concern with no responsibility, but He cares *for* us. 1 Peter 5:7 says, ". . . casting all your care on Him, *for He cares for you.*" I am grateful that God is not only concerned about me, but that He takes full responsibility for my welfare, my health, my life, and for providing not only for my physical needs, but also for my spiritual and emotional needs. Along with all of that, He provides me with a life-giving relationship with Him.

He tells us to ". . . come boldly unto the throne of grace, that we might obtain mercy, and find grace to help in time of need" (Hebrews 4:16 KJV). My boldness has grown in the past six months and so has my capacity to cast my cares on Him. I am better at receiving His grace, as well as understanding and trusting that God truly cares *for* His children. I am grateful that His supply of grace and care, as well as healthy blood cells, never runs dry.

Saturday, June 21 — Heading Toward the Goal with Him

I returned to the lab yesterday for blood tests. My WBC count was only up to 6, when last round it was 13.5. I was not encouraged, but the nurse told me that she was pleased that they are increasing.

This week, I told a friend that "arriving" is not our main goal in our spiritual life. The important issue is that we are on the right path, headed toward the goal. Now I have a real and practical example.

Salvation is only the starting line — not the finish line. Growing in the Lord is a daily process that He calls "working out our salvation" (see Philippians 2:12). Sometimes that "working out" involves our falling down and getting up again or making wrong decisions and getting off the path so that He has to guide us back to where we need to be. As we daily seek Him — studying His Word and talking with (not at) Him in prayer — He guides us. We will not arrive at our goal until the day we get to heaven. I am finding joy and encouragement in walking through the process knowing that I will one day finish the journey. He promises that He will complete the good work He has begun in me (Philippians 1:6). I am grateful.

Therefore, rather than be discouraged with my WBC, I am encouraged that the cells are growing in the right direction.

Also, this morning, I noticed that Wasco was limping. I picked him up and tried to look at the hurt paw, but he bit my hand. I thought about how often our pain governs our responses. When we are in pain, we often resist help from the One who can heal us. He is the healer (Isaiah 53:5; 1 Peter 2:24). How grateful I am for the Lord's hand on me. I am persevering and cooperating with the healing process.

Thursday, June 26 — Pulling up the Roots

I felt good enough this week to work in the garden for a little while. I think God loves gardens. His first discourses with man and woman were in a garden (Genesis 1:28–29), and He always speaks to me there. I love working outside because I know the garden is a place where He will speak to my heart. I go there with eager anticipation.

If you've ever had a garden, you know it involves much work. With the spring rain and now the heat and sunshine, our garden is growing. We have tomatoes, jalapeños, bell peppers and potatoes. The cucumbers, squash, and cantaloupes, corn and okra are growing. But, as the plants have flourished, so have the weeds! Our garden covers nearly one-fourth acre, so we have a lot of plants and even more weeds.

Because of my limited energy, I have not regularly weeded the garden. Yesterday, I decided to at least pull the weeds around the plants, so the plants could get nourishment. But when you pull weeds, you have to get the roots. If the roots remain, the weeds are only pruned and grow back, sometimes even stronger.

As I was pulling weeds, I thought about the "spiritual weeds' in my heart — the reoccurring fears and doubts that have surfaced throughout my life—and I realized that they return because I never dealt with the roots.

We try to make ourselves look good on the outside, as we will do just about anything to keep from having to dig deep in our lives to get rid of our bad attitudes, including ignoring or denying them. Yet the attitudes keep surfacing because the roots are still there.

One day, Charlie was talking with a neighbor about plowing our pastures. Charlie has a plow that goes on the back of our tractor. The man said that our plow would only dig up the top three to four inches of soil. He said that would not greatly improve the crops. Charlie needs a "deep plow" that digs deep in the soil and brings buried roots and rocks to the surface. The man said, "We call that a *repentance* plow!"

During the past six months, God has used His "deep plow" to deal with some root issues in my life and bring me to repentance. Many of those attitudes I learned from my parents, who learned them from their parents—generational issues that I do not want to pass on to my children. Many were lies that I have believed about myself and God. Some were just bad attitudes that I have justified through the years.

I can more easily see the "weeds" in someone else's life than my own. However, I am only responsible for my own attitudes, so have determined to keep my focus on my own life. I want to grow in the spiritual fruit God wants for me: compassion, understanding, love, kindness, patience, long-suffering. The desire of my heart is to look more like Him. I am thankful that *the Lord wants us to be free of things that He has not planted in our lives*, and He is willing to use His truth to work deep into the soil of our hearts to set us free from the weeds and the roots (John 8:32).

I am feeling good this week and even had the energy to teach at church last night. My next chemotherapy session is next week—and the process continues. In the meantime, I am enjoying the strength and lack of pain and nausea. I even had Mexican food this week! God is faithful and you have been too. Thank you!

✄ *GUEST*

Your journal is such an inspiration to me and helps through the difficulty I am facing. Sometimes, I am running on the path, sometimes walking, sometimes crawling, but I am on the right path, always calling out to Jesus to help me and clinging to Him when all seems dark. At times, I feel that I am on this path with no one beside me and I long for encouragement. Your honest sharing has been the encouragement I need. Thanks so much. I am reminded of the Scripture that tells us that in our weakness He is strong (2 Corinthians 12:9-10). It seems backwards to us but that is what God does; He shows His power in our weakness. Praise the Lord for this amazing truth!

Much love to you, my dear friend,

Sharon

℥ GUEST

Lots of wisdom as you write about gardening and root issues. For a moment, I was feeling a little smug about seeing the weeds in someone else's life. . . . Thanks for straightening me out. We should praise the Lord when we see our weeds so we can get at the root. I have noticed that some weeds are harder to uproot than others — some are so resistant!

The Lord be praised for surely He has you in the palm of His protective hand and His wonderful Grace.

Darleen

Sunday, June 29 — Finishing Strong

Yesterday, I went with Carie, Rebekah, and Nathaniel to Waco to get Elisabeth after a week long band camp at Baylor University. We were there for the youth concert and I was amazed at how middle-school musicians sounded so excellent. What a treat.

On the way, Rebekah said she was writing a story, and she read to me what she had written. I could envision what she was writing about, as her words were so descriptive. Her writing was wonderful. Then she made the statement that she had the beginnings of many stories at home, but that she didn't finish very many of them. Her statement reminded me of the many projects I have started and not finished. A close friend once asked me to go into business with her, and our job would be to finish other people's unfinished projects. Charlie said that I could do that as soon as I had finished all of my projects. We never formed that business! Soon afterward, I got rid of many partially completed projects. That was freeing.

As I consider the process of healing and going through chemotherapy, I have thought that the closer I came to the end, the easier it would be. However, as I approached the halfway point, the treatment did not get easier. Now as I look at two treatments remaining, a battle is raging inside of me, and the next few months seem like they will never end. For some reason, the process has become more difficult.

If all of my tests are within proper range, I will receive treatment five on Tuesday. I could easily quit today and walk away. Perhaps that is because the last three weeks were such a challenge.

As I have talked with the Lord about this, He reminded me of a message that I shared at a pastors' revival meeting in Japan. The message was titled, "Finishing Strong."

I find that it is easy to "start strong." We set goals. We are especially good at that on January 1. However, we rarely persevere and often don't finish, much less finish with the strength and dedication that we had when we began.

The Scriptures provide many examples. King Saul, Israel's first King, was anointed by God. However, he eventually disobeyed to the point that, out of fear of the people, he usurped the place of the priests and offered the sacrifice. He rejected the Word of God. As a result, God said that He regretted making Saul king and God removed His presence from Saul (1 Samuel 15). Saul's life ended tragically as he committed suicide.

King Solomon began strong. God asked him what he wanted, and Solomon asked for wisdom to rule the people in a righteous manner. God not only blessed him with wisdom but also gave him more riches than any other king in history. Solomon loved the Lord and obeyed Him. People came from all over the world to meet Solomon because of His reputation for wisdom and riches. However, in the end, his heart was turned to the idols of his foreign wives. He started strong but Solomon died under God's anger. The kingdom was torn out of his hand (1 Kings 3:3-14; 11:11).

Many others are listed in the Scriptures, and even many more not listed there, some of whom we personally know, who have started strong but along the way they stopped seeking God. They turned away because the price for Godliness was too much to pay. They quit serving God.

I understand the temptation to quit what we have set out to accomplish when the way is too difficult. I have been praying and seeking the Lord about this. During worship this morning, we sang a song that said God will not relent until He has all of my heart. I held onto that word and wept with hope. I want to accomplish all He has for me, but even more, I want His character to be formed in me. I trust Him to finish the good work He has begun in me (Philippians 1:6). I am not afraid of what would happen physically if I quit the treatments, but I do not want to miss something in the spiritual realm, which can only come through my obedience to see this through to the end. I want to finish and I want to *finish strong*.

Charlie and I had the privilege of hearing Steve Fry speak this morning. He is an amazing composer, author, worship leader, and teacher. He said,

> Persevering is a way of life for the Christian. We must learn to completely depend on Jesus here, on this earth. We live a lifestyle of enduring and must have "holy tenacity." Do not look for the end of the struggle, but look for the Lord in the midst of the struggle (Worship Conference, Plano, TX, June 29, 2008).

As I consider whether to go forward, I have no choice. I have counted the cost, which God says to do (Luke 14:28). And, even though the price seems high, the price for quitting is even greater and one I am not willing to pay.

As I seek to persevere, I am thankful for you, my friends and family in the Body of Christ. Thank you for your faith and passion for Jesus and for being faithful to pray on my behalf. I am grateful for each time you have spoken truth into my life and have brought encouragement and even conviction to my heart. Thank you for not praying, "God, *if* you can . . ." but for believing the Word of God, calling on God with faith, and standing with authority against the enemy.

I do not fear that God will fail to come through. He is trustworthy and faithful. But I am often afraid that I will fail Him; I am keenly aware of my weaknesses. Please continue to pray for my endurance, and that I will rely totally on His Holy Spirit. Pray that I will do this with great joy. When this is over, I want to hear Him say, "Well done."

❧ GUEST

I chuckled as I read about the business of finishing unfinished projects.

We do agree with your prayer request to stay the course in victory because God is upholding you. . . . Through Him, you shall do valiantly. I think of Psalm 18 as I read your journal. . . . He is our Strength, our Rock, our Fortress, and our Deliverer. Thank God that we can do all things through Christ who strengthens us . . . and He always causes us to triumph in Christ Jesus.

As we worshiped this morning, I reflected on Colossians 2:9–10 (AMP):

> For in Him the whole fullness of Deity (the Godhead) continues to dwell in bodily form [giving complete expression of the divine nature]. And you are in Him, made full and having come to fullness of life [in Christ you too are filled with the Godhead — Father, Son and Holy Spirit — and reach full spiritual stature]. And He is the Head of all rule and authority [of every angelic principality and power].

That settles it. Christ alone is our hope of glory. I find myself being able to do things that I used to feel guilty for not doing, because I have concentrated more on Him and less on my lack. I endeavor to concentrate on who I am *in Him*. . . .

I love you so much and especially appreciate the issues of life that you share.

Darleen

❧ GUEST

Hollis and I agree with you that finishing strong is the challenge . . . that we are aligning with Him and He is the plumb line. You have our prayers and love, for Suzanne, finishing strong is His sanctifying delight, and we never know just how He does it, but He does it.

Love you more than Blue Bell® ice cream.

C J

I received treatment 5 yesterday. Last night was a challenge — a few complications, but I got through it. Today, I went back to the doctor for the WBC booster shot, which should take effect in the next few days. I am getting ready to take a nap, which is still a strange event for me during the middle of the day.

On the way to the doctor this morning, I shared with Charlie something that made me laugh. Life on this earth is sometimes depicted in Scripture as "running the race." That idea takes on a very different picture today as just getting one foot in front of the other is the goal; that is not exactly what I picture as "running." I can imagine myself as the tortoise rather than the hare, but the tortoise did win the race in the end.

I read about a marathon runner who went to the Olympics in 1968. He quickly discovered that he was not as fast as the other runners, and he was injured in the race. When he finally came into the arena, everyone else had long since crossed the finish line, and most of the people remaining in the arena were workers cleaning up after the race. When he crossed the finish line, someone asked why he didn't quit. His answer was, "My country did not send me to Mexico City to start the race. They sent me to finish".[25] What perseverance.

I am grateful that for many of the races that we run and the challenges that we face, we are not in a competition. *The race is within us and is for building our character.*

I continue to run this race slowly, one step, one day, one event at a time. God's grace is amazing and sufficient as I rest in Him. And as several of you have reminded me, He will carry me when I cannot do the running. He truly is faithful, as are you, His servants. Blessings to each of you.

❧ GUEST

You know how the "race" imagery is directly touching me, and I appreciate your sharing how God is speaking to you through this. The race *does* become more difficult the closer we get to the finish line, but we must push on.

I don't know if I ever told you about my first (and only) 10K race. I decided to run the Columbus 10K in 2000. I ran a good race . . . for me. The race was two 5K (3.1-mile) circles on the same course.

I ran the first half in about 25 minutes, and as I came to the start and finish line, the crowds began to scream and yell and point at me. I wondered why. Then, about 100 feet from the line, a VERY fast runner passed me on the left . . . and won the race. Everyone was watching him and me because we were crossing the same line, but I still had half of the race to run!

I kept running, even though all of the cheering people at the sidewalks were gone and the water tables were cleared. I was so slow. I had to remember that the point for me was not to win the race but to FINISH the race. I kept running and singing and praying and trying to endure. About 0.5K from the finish line, a cooled-off runner walked past me on the sidewalk, turned around, and began running with me, cheering me on and telling me how close I was to finishing. But for that man, I might have quit the race, but he was so encouraging that I charged on and knew: *I could do this!* (Lord, to this day, please bless that man!)

I finished the 10K in 58 minutes, the last finisher of the Columbus 10K. But I finished!

Your race may get more difficult at the end, but we are here to cheer you on and remind you that you are close to the end and, in God's strength, *you can do this!*

Love you SO much and am so proud of how you reflect God's glory and grace!

Carie

⚜ GUEST

As we press on in the path before us, may we ever intercede for those whose race is not directed toward the Kingdom of God. Everyone's race will take him somewhere. May our goal be holiness as we pursue God.

Dianna

A couple of weeks ago I had to tie our tomato plants to stakes because the plants are loaded with tomatoes, and some of the plants were on the ground because they were so heavy.

Those tomato plants reminded me of God's children. We sometimes have the idea that as we grow and mature, we can stand alone. Yet, as these tomato plants grow bigger and mature, producing fruit, they must have something to "lean on." Otherwise, they will fall on the ground where the bugs can easily get them, or they break under the weight of the fruit.

Even as Christians, we often think maturity means independence — that we can "go it alone" and that we need other people less. Our American attitude and independent spirit encourage this. However, the opposite is true. After all, His ways are not our ways (Isaiah 55:8–9). Our independent spirit is never healthy. When we believe we do not need the support of other Christians, we are open to falling on the ground and having our roots attach to the earth (the world) or we can simply break down.

The word "bear," as in "bear one another's burdens" (Galatians 6:2 NASB), is a picture of a gardener's stake holding up a plant. To "bear" means "to carry, to support, to keep from falling"[26].The stake carries part of the weight of the mature plant with fruit. Bearing one another's burdens is the relationship we as Christians are to have with each other.

In Exodus 17:8–13, Joshua was on the battlefield, and Moses was on a hill overlooking the fight. As long as Moses held up the rod of God, the children of Israel would win. But when Moses' arms tired and he lowered the rod, the children of Israel began to lose. Therefore, Aaron and Hur stood on either side of Moses and held his arms, and the battle was won. They "staked" up his arms, and he rested on their strength.

I can often feel the arms of others holding me up when I get weary. Every prayer and word of encouragement is like those arms, holding me up and motivating me to keep on moving forward. I know this battle is going to be won.

A practical example of this principle was demonstrated many years ago when I was going to a women's conference and wanted a friend to go with me. She would not because she always got sick when riding a bus. Three of us committed to pray that if she would go, she would not get sick. She agreed to go, and we prayed. She never got sick. However, each of us got slightly nauseous. I learned through that event what it is like to actually carry another person's burden. That experience also helped my understanding of Jesus literally bearing our sins on the cross (1 Peter 2:24). His "carrying" was real, not symbolic.

The closer we get to the Lord, the more we realize we can do nothing on our own and without Him. And the closer I get to Him, the more I realize how little I actually know about Him. We cannot grasp the eternal nature of who He is. That is why He sent Jesus to identify with us and to reveal God to us (Colossians 1:19).

And He created us to need each other. That has been obvious to me the past six months. I would not be walking this journey in the way I am if I were doing this alone. Your support is holding me up. Some of those who are praying for and encouraging me are people whom I have never met. Yet, their hearts were touched by God, and they are ministering to me. As much as I am aware of my need for other members of the Body of Christ, I am also aware of my accountability to them, and I have a sense of responsibility to walk as Jesus would walk through this situation.

I taught at church a couple of weeks ago and shared that what we do affects others in the Body of Christ because we are connected. In the physical realm, when one part of our physical body breaks down or hurts, it affects our entire body. I am experiencing that in the natural realm. The same is true in the spiritual realm because God says we are connected. We are *one body* with Christ as the head (Romans 12; 1 Corinthians 12).

The Body of Christ is not just a pile of body parts. That would be a dismembered body and would have no life. We as His Body are connected and filled with life. Part of the Body is in heaven — the "great cloud of witnesses" (Hebrews 12:1) — and part of the Body is all over the earth. This is not an easy concept to grasp, because we do not personally know all those parts and we rarely feel like part of something that big. But God says we are connected (1 Corinthians 12:12–27) and we are to accept His word by faith even when we cannot see or feel it.

We are told to pray for others with the same intensity and urgency as if we were going through their situation ourselves. We are to consider ourselves connected with every Christian — even those around the world.

My prayer is that each of you will know and embrace that oneness and support of Christ and of His Body, even without having to go through crisis. May the Lord work in us so we encourage others constantly, letting them know that each of us is a necessary and valuable part of something much bigger. (Many of you already do that!)

Lord, please give us the strategic picture. Give us Your wisdom so we can see things as You do and have deeper understanding and deeper love for Your Body.

Tuesday, July 8 — Living Life from the Inside

Yesterday, Nathaniel saw me without my wig and said, "Grammy, you look like an alien!" That was a *huge* compliment, and he said it with such awe.

I went to the lab for blood tests yesterday. My WBC count was very low, and I was running a fever. The doctor put me on antibiotics and told me to come back on Wednesday rather than Thursday.

The past week had been challenging. Tuesday through Thursday, I slept and rested most of the time. On Thursday, the pain set in, either from chemotherapy or from the WBC booster shot; I am not sure which. The pain is a strange kind of pain that I had not experienced until chemotherapy. When that pain comes, my skin hurts, starting with my bald head. I can feel the pain in my muscles and even in my bones. My teeth and eyeballs hurt. I struggle to sit down because I hurt when anything touches my body. Lying on the bed or wearing clothes hurts.

The pain increased from Thursday noon through Sunday. Then Sunday evening about 9 p.m., I was sitting in my study, and it was like a cloud lifted off my body, and most of the pain was gone in a matter of seconds. I took time to praise and rejoice.

Some people ask me how many treatments I have to go. I rejoice that I am scheduled for only one more. But I cannot see that far ahead. The treatment is not the main issue. The weeks of painful side effects that follow the treatment are the hard part. I am still working through treatment five and have more than two weeks to go.

Things always look very different when I am walking through them than when I am an observer. That is certainly true with facing cancer and the treatments. During a crisis, time concepts change; it seems to move in slow motion. I suspect that for many people, the past six months have gone very fast, but for me, the year has already been long. At the same time, it has been fruitful and beneficial.

More often than not, things look different from the "inside" than they look from the "outside." Our hearts look different from the inside. We are often sad when our intent was to encourage someone and our words did not convey our heart or we were misunderstood. On the other hand, we can easily miss our own blind spots, bad attitudes, and bitterness, which we justify and excuse, while others are very aware of those attitudes.

We also know that the church looks different from the inside than it does from the outside. The Body of Christ is often viewed as people who follow religious rules of dos and don'ts and who are judgmental, hypocritical, and politically incorrect. And if you happen to admit that you hear God's voice, they believe you are crazy.

But on the inside, we know the love, warmth, and fellowship, not only of the Lord but of the saints who stand with us in our passion for God and for His will to be done. We know the comfort of hearing His voice speak to our hearts, assuring us that we belong to Him and that He knows and loves us. In the midst of our lives, with "inside" and "outside" perspectives and how things are not always as they seem to be, I am grateful that we know the One who knows everything in detail and who sees the reality and truth of how things *are*, rather than the way they appear to be. God says He does not see things as man does. He does not look at the outside, but He looks at the heart (1 Samuel 16:7).

How thankful I am for His all-seeing and all-knowing ability. Were it not for His amazing love, mercy, and grace, I would not be able to endure the concept of His knowing my heart, my attitudes, and my deepest desires. He knows even what we cannot put into thoughts or communicate in words. He knows things we do not see. He knows things we do not want to see. He knows and He cares. He knows what it will take to heal us and to set us free.

As we seek Him and lay our hearts before Him, He is there and knows what we need (Matthew 6:8) and is even answering our prayers before we ask. I am *so* grateful—for Him, and for you and your support.

⚘ GUEST

Isaiah 43:1–5 (NASB)

> But now, thus says the Lord, your Creator, O Jacob, And He who formed you, O Israel, "Do not fear, for I have redeemed you; I have called you by name; you are Mine! When you pass through the waters, I will be with you; And through the rivers, they will not overflow you. When you walk through the fire, you will not be

scorched, Nor will the flame burn you. For I am the Lord your God, The Holy One of Israel, your Savior; I have given Egypt as your ransom, Cush and Seba in your place. *Since* you are precious in My sight, Since you are honored and I love you, I will give *other* men in your place and *other* peoples in exchange for your life. Do not fear, for I am with you . . .."

Love you and am praying for you and Daddy constantly!

Christie

Monday, July 14—Learning from Each Other

Many years ago, I heard the story of blind men who were describing an elephant as they were feeling different parts of the animal. They each had a unique perspective—no two descriptions were alike. They were simply analyzing the elephant by feeling different parts of the animal's body, whether the leg, tusk, tail, ear, trunk, or the enormous side that seemed to have no end. Who was correct? Of course, we know they were all correct. And the only way to get an accurate perspective of what the elephant looks like is to put all those pieces together.

When I was a new Christian. I thought I knew everything, and I told everyone all I knew. Like those blind men, what I knew was true but actually turned out to be very little. The closer we get to God, we begin to get a different perspective and are overwhelmed by His enormity and majesty. Also, the closer we come to Him, we taste that sweetness of intimate fellowship with Him as Savior, friend, protector, and lover of our souls.

The more I know of God, the more I realize just how little I do know about Him. This year, I have questioned and experienced areas in my life that I've never seen before. I have learned things about Him that I didn't know or only had "head knowledge" but no experiential knowledge. He has not yet failed to meet me at the place of need and to give revelation of Himself, which brought peace back to my life along with a new depth of understanding.

When we are with other Christians who have a different perspective and different theology about God, we do not need to be intimidated. We can learn from them and hear testimony of things of God that we have not yet experienced. We must measure all things according to the Scriptures, but I have learned many precious things about God from my Catholic, Baptist, Methodist, Episcopal, and evangelical friends—from those who have a different perspective. As with the blind men, none of us has the total picture of who God is. For example, I never understood or appreciated liturgy until we were in a military chapel. As I sat through liturgical services, I found an understanding of God that I had never known before. And I learned the value of repentance and communion from my Catholic friends.

As Christians, together we are the one Body of Christ, even with our different perspectives, and we can learn from each other. I look forward to the day when we will all worship together in Heaven, without labels and walls to separate us.

Also, as the situations of my life change, I become like the different blind men. Each time I am in a different situation, I experience a different aspect of God's character. A crisis can be the very catalyst that drives us closer and deeper into His presence and allows us to experience His different attributes. This was true about King David as throughout the Psalms he cried out to God in the midst of his challenging circumstances.

Presently, I am learning perseverance, and I am so grateful that the Spirit of God is long-suffering. I continually ask Him to be in control of my life. I pray for patience and endurance. These attributes are not part of my human nature. But my desire is that the Lord will build them into my life and replace any impatience, apathy, and procrastination.

Another thing I have been focusing on is how to be pleasing and acceptable to God. Too often, I have considered what I could do for Him or looked at the situations of my life and judged whether I was measuring up. However, I am not the one who decides if I am pleasing God. He sets the rules!

Recently, I have talked to people who are walking through crises and have learned that many of them struggle with being pleasing and acceptable to God when they feel worthless and are unable to serve Him the way they are accustomed. God has made it very clear that for us to please Him, we must come to Him and put our faith in Him—believing that He exists and that He rewards those who diligently seek Him. In Hebrews 11:6, it says that without faith it is impossible to please God. That has nothing to do with whether we are sick or well, rich or poor, or if our lives are going smoothly or we are in a battle. In every situation, He can be trusted. He invites us to seek Him—with the promise that we *will* find Him, even in our present situation (Matthew 7:7-8); that He will never leave us (Hebrews 13:5); and that He will use all things for the good of His children (Romans 8:28). That includes even our worst situations and the things the enemy brings to steal, kill, and destroy us (John 10:10).

If you are walking in a difficult situation, you have an opportunity to learn something new about God—about His amazing character and His faithfulness. You too can come closer to Him as you seek Him and trust that He will reward you with more of Himself. He is Life.

The closer I get to the end of treatments, the more I know that I cannot run this race alone. Thank you for faithfully continuing to run alongside me. I am grateful for that most valuable and precious gift of your prayers. God *does* hear and *is* answering.

✤ GUEST

I was surprised when I read your entry for today, because I had one of those "I know so little about God" experiences yesterday. Isn't it amazing that even though we know so little about Him, He knows everything about us?

Carie

Friday, July 18 — Celebrating Every Day of Life

I had a birthday this week and I had fun. Birthdays have taken on a new meaning and value this year. I love that the American Cancer Society says it is the "official sponsor of birthdays".[27] That makes me smile. At times, I didn't like growing older. Now, I realize that growing older is a gift, and I prefer it to the possibility of not growing older!

In the past, I have not been into big celebrations for my birthday. I did celebrate my 46th year, but that is a story for a different time. And the girls gave me a wonderful party when I celebrated 60 years, as it was a milestone in my life. Otherwise, I usually prefer to have an ordinary day and to spend time with family. I do sometimes stretch out the celebration for a week or so by going to lunch with friends.

This year, I have a different perspective of my birthday, and I will probably celebrate more exuberantly with each birthday for the rest of my life. When you face the possibility of not having more birthdays, each one becomes more precious. Actually, each day becomes more valuable, and I am grateful for the gift of life, even on days when I hurt or feel bad. Even the pain reminds me that I am alive.

At the oncologist's office, I have met many people with "terminal cancer" who do not know how much longer they have to live. The truth is, as I have found out firsthand this year, none of us knows when life will end. My greatest fear when I faced the diagnosis of cancer was that I would die without having completed all that God has called me to do.

I know what Paul means when he says that to be with Christ is gain. To live in Heaven with Christ is the goal of my life and has been since 1970, when I surrendered my life to Jesus and asked Him to be my Savior and Lord and when His Holy Spirit moved into me. For the past 38 years, my focus has been to prepare for eternity by seeking to become what He wants me to be, to become more like Him, and to share with others who Jesus is. I want every person to know the blessing of a love relationship with God through Jesus Christ.

While I want to be with Him, I do not want to go before God calls me home. I still have things to do on earth. My destiny is not complete, and I want to accomplish those things that He has set apart for me.

On the day when He calls me home, I don't want to say what I often say to Charlie, "Could you wait a minute? I haven't quite finished what I'm doing. . . . Are we going to be late?" Therefore, I am working at overcoming procrastination and at being diligently obedient and timely in what God has told me to do.

I pray that you, too, are celebrating life this day, and that you are busy doing what God has called you to do. Today is a gift that God has given to each of us. Our gift to Him is how we use this day for His glory. He spoke each of us into being; we were fearfully and wonderfully made, and His hand is still upon us (Psalm 139). May we walk fully and wholeheartedly according to His plans with rejoicing and celebration — until promotion day when He calls us home.

❧ GUEST

Good morning, Suzanne, and happy birthday. Sometimes, when I read your blog, I feel like I am intruding on some powerful love talk. . . . His koinonia (fellowship) is life, and we rejoice exceedingly over all that you and others are writing.

Yesterday, as I was in our garden, I noticed how this year's garden is different from other years'. Our garden has flourished—not with fruit but with blossoms. I counted 15 blossoms on one squash plant, and that plant has not borne any fruit. Then, the Lord began to speak to me. We love blossoms but sometimes fall short on fruit, or we settle for blossoms and won't go the extra mile for fruit. The Lord reminded me that we are known by our fruit.

As all this cruised through my heart, I thought of you, and the fruit that is laden all around you. We rejoice in the 38 years you have chosen to be about the Father's business. I like that you not only love to divide the Word, but you also love to live the Word. I know that as a fact. (I hear that also in your husband and children's entries, as well as your friends.)

I suppose that we become more pensive as we age, so what a gift of God we have to meditate in His presence. What was meant to do harm, God has so turned to good in you, reaping deeper truths and greater appreciation . . . and outright exultation that is extreme joy!

C J

Monday, July 21 — *Praying for a Miracle*

Shortly after I became a Christian, I developed a hunger for reading the Bible. I was amazed at things that were written there, as well as being surprised at many things that were not written in the Bible. I had heard and lived by many proverbs as I grew up, such as "God helps those who help themselves," "The quickest way to a man's heart is through his stomach," and "Pretty is as pretty does." I couldn't find those in the Scriptures! But, as I read, I was captivated by the miracles that *were recorded* in the Bible. One day, I told the Lord, "If the early church had depended on me to spread the Gospel and to show the world who You are, it would have died within weeks. I am not living the way Your followers lived. Lord, at all costs, change my life!"

I felt a huge gap between my life and the lives of God's people recorded in history. I was not experiencing miracles in my life, and I didn't know people who were. I began to pray that God would make me like the Christians in the book of Acts.

In the mid-1970s, I began to see the answers to that prayer. First, we began to meet people who shared their experiences of Biblical miracles. Our faith began to grow. Then, Charlie and I found ourselves experiencing God's amazing miracles. I was physically healed several times and delivered of addictions. We prayed for people whom the Lord instantly delivered or healed, some who had been diagnosed with terminal diseases. God began doing miracles in our finances, and other unusual things began to happen. For example, the four of us ate daily from the same cereal box for almost a month, and it did not empty, and the milk did not spoil or run out until payday! One day, I thought the car was broken because I had driven for a week and the gas gauge had not moved. Gasoline was being rationed and we could only purchase gas on certain days. Charlie took the car to the gas station and attempted to put more gas in the tank, only to find the car was still completely full. We shared this with our pastor who reminded us with examples from the Scriptures that God does these kinds of things (see 1 Kings 17:14; Matthew 14:19-20).

Vine's Dictionary provides two Greek words for the English word "miracle." One word means "a wonder or a sign of divine authority." The other word in Greek is "dunamis," which is the same as that for "power" and is the word from which we get the word "dynamite." "Miracle" is defined as "works of a supernatural origin and character, such as could not be produced by natural agents and means".[28]

When I was diagnosed with cancer, many people prayed for a miracle. We did not see the instant healing for which we asked. We knew God could do that, but He did not. Instead, He has done many smaller miracles — that is, if any miracle can be considered as small. The size of miracles are only in the eyes of man.

The Lord spoke to Charlie in early February through the story where Jesus told Peter to go out to the deep water and cast his nets. Peter had been fishing all night and had not caught anything, but he obeyed Jesus, and his nets came up full of fish, so full that the nets began to break. In the beginning of that story, Peter addressed Jesus as Master of the ship. However, after catching all those fish, Peter called Jesus "Lord and Master of all." His perspective of Jesus changed because of the miracle. That section of Scripture ends saying they "left everything and followed Him" (Luke 5:1–11 NASB).

Peter did not catch one big whale, but the miracle was in the many small fish. The Lord showed Charlie that He was going to do the same in my life through the healing process: I was not going to have a big instantaneous healing, but I was going to experience many miracles along the way. And it has happened.

From the beginning, I had the assurance that God was going to heal me, though not instantly. Healing comes in many forms. My healing is coming through a process and is taking time. I think of the woman whom Jesus instantly healed of internal bleeding (Mark 5:24–34). She had suffered pain, ill health, rejection, and loneliness for 12 long years. I wonder if she called it an "instant" healing.

God is bigger and far more powerful than the finite ways of the world that He created, and I am always excited to see how He works. Miracles are demonstrated throughout the Scriptures, from Genesis to Revelation. I have seen healings and miracles, which are what I'm requesting when I pray, "Your kingdom come. Your will be done on earth as it is in heaven." (Matthew 6:10 NKJV). I have seen people give their lives to Christ after He worked a miracle in their lives. They want to know a God who loves them that much.

Changing lives — spiritually, emotionally, physically, and in every other way — is something that God seems to love doing, and each change is a miracle. At the same time, I know that my focus must remain on Him, His Word, and His character, rather than on His works, His methods, or His timing. His works flow out of who He is, but are not a replacement for our knowing Him personally and becoming like Him. We must follow Him. In the process, we come to know Him as Lord and Master of all creation as well as of our lives.

When the Lord said I would receive daily miracles, I began praying that I would have spiritual eyes to see what He was doing. And He has given me vision, wisdom, and a heart to see many things He has done. Often when His miracles are recorded, the Scripture first says, "He was moved with compassion." Jesus' works flowed out of His love for people. The power of His love changed lives. It still does. Many times the miracles we experience come under the world's labels of chance, coincidence, luck, or fate, but they are actually God's love gifts to us and opportunities for us to see that He is at work on our behalf.

As Charlie prays for us at the end of the day, He thanks the Lord for all the things that we have seen God do during the day. Then, He thanks the Lord for all the things He has done that we have not seen. I rejoice that we can trust our Heavenly Father to be working, protecting, and moving in our lives and on our behalf, even when we do not see what He is doing.

I pray that you too have eyes to see His power at work in your life, as He overcomes the natural realm with His miracles. Every time I see His hand move, I have cause to celebrate and rejoice!

༅ GUEST

One of my favorite quotes is from Elizabeth Barrett Browning:

> Earth's crammed with heaven,
> And every common bush afire with God;
> But only he who sees, takes off his shoes,
> The rest sit round it and pluck blackberries . . .[29]

God is everywhere: in our celebration, in our sorrow. He is in the midst of the big—the obvious—the trumpets blowing—kind of miracles, and He is in the midst of the small—the common—daily miracles. We miss a lot about Him when we overlook His involvement in the small details of our lives. Those are the intimate moments with Him, when you see Him move in the "ordinary" things and make the extraordinary out of it.

Thanks for reminding us of these truths, Mom, and for encouraging each of us to press into Christ and to cling to His character.

Christie

༅ GUEST

I love your post today. You and I have talked about the little miracles that God does and how we need to be grateful for those just as much as we are for the big miracles. I've often prayed that God would provide me with a big miracle in my life, but as I look back over the last eight or nine years, I realize that every day can be a little miracle from God that keeps me in His will and reminds me to walk in faith.

I wish God had given us a big miracle and healed you of cancer with no treatment, but then I realize how many people you would not have met and touched, and I realize that God used this disease (Satan's plan) for His glory and for many big and little miracles.

Who am I to judge these miracles or to define what seems little to me as insignificant?

Your attitude through this has been a big miracle. Thank you for your transparent sharing of your struggles and victories and your giving God praise for all He has done.

Carie

Wednesday, July 23 — Completing the Course with Treatment Six

Last Sunday at church, the congregation broke into small groups to pray. The man next to me began to pray for us to have dedication and perseverance. He mentioned 2 Kings 13:14-19 when Elisha told King Jehoash that if he struck the ground with his arrows, he would destroy the enemy's army. Jehoash struck the ground only three times and then stopped. The prophet was angry and said if he had continued and struck the ground five or six times, Jehoash would have completely destroyed the enemy, but because he stopped, he would not have total victory.

I wonder what causes us to persevere. I was thinking again today how easy it is to begin strong, but finishing with determination and passion is often a challenge.

Recently, I told Charlie that I wanted to quit chemotherapy. I did not think I could go through the rest of the treatments. I knew I could not quit; I had to persevere. But continuing was a huge struggle. I feel it is significant that this week I will have treatment six. I am striking the ground for the sixth time, and I believe I will have total victory and complete healing. Hearing about Jehoash was divine timing and gave me strength to persevere. I had never met the man who shared the Scripture, and this situation was obviously arranged by God.

I do know that the ability and endurance to finish treatment has not been accomplished by my own strength. Your prayers and encouragement have helped to keep me moving forward. The past few weeks have been a battle, in many ways other than just physically. I have not been able to see "the end" ahead as I have walked through each day with its challenges. Only in the past few days, I finally have anticipation that this season of life will actually end. I must still walk in patience, knowing that this last treatment may have a longer and stronger impact. Then, my body will begin the slow process of rebuilding, and I pray I will return to normal energy and wellness.

My joy is not only in finishing chemotherapy but also in the perseverance that has allowed me to complete the process and to obtain victory. I am grateful for God's amazing grace and faithfulness. My heart is filled with joy that I am heading toward the finish line.

Tomorrow, I will have my last chemotherapy treatment. So far, I still have some eyebrows and eyelashes, though I hear that they will probably disappear in the next few weeks. I also still have fingernails, and even though they are in bad condition, I am praying that I keep them. (I sit under a blanket, freezing, with my hands in ice through the treatment because this can help me keep my fingernails.)

Last Friday, I had the first "last!" I went to the nuclear medicine laboratory for my last heart scan. Then I began to realize that this process will end. I will not miss the blood tests and shots and scans, but I will miss the people who work in those clinics. Those people have blessed me. The same is true about the people in the oncologist's office. The employees there always smile and encourage me. When I asked Holly, the technician who administers my treatment, how she can always be in a good mood, she answered that her calling in life is to help people get well, and she loves doing it. Her attitude lights up that treatment room, and her smile and gentleness make a difference in the patients' lives.

I know that when this process ends, I will never be the same again. What I have experienced has altered my perspective such that I will not return to the same thinking and same approach to life that I had before January. And I don't want to return to the "old way" of thinking. I am thankful for the changes in my attitudes and my perspectives of life, and I want to spend the rest of my life helping other people to walk through crisis situations.

I will always be grateful for the way each of you have continued to walk with me. I want to walk with others in that same way, encouraging them through the process. I pray the Lord's blessings on each of you.

I would appreciate your prayers tomorrow and especially in the weeks following. Carie said the last treatment is usually the most difficult, mostly due to the accumulation of chemicals that causes more intense side effects. I will update you after tomorrow.

. . . I was thinking this morning about the desert through which you have walked with oases along the way. You have appreciated them, not allowing the surrounding desert to be all you have seen. May we all see and appreciate God's blessings in the hard times and remember that He has higher purposes, that He who began a good work will also finish it.

I love you and Charlie.

Praying on,
Dianna

⁂ GUEST

My sister-in-law said your journal encouraged her today. She had considered telling the doctors to forget the chemo, but she will keep on keeping on. She also said that calcium (even cheap calcium tablets from the drug store) dissolved in ice water will keep your nails even stronger. . . .

We will be praying special prayers tomorrow.

Much love,
Darleen

Friday, July 25 — Experiencing the First of the Lasts

I went to bed Wednesday night with some of that old familiar dread looming over me. I rested some but never slept, so I was very tired when I got up Thursday morning for an early appointment. However, by breakfast time, I could sense that people were praying for me. My life was so saturated in grace that I had no fear or dread and was excited about possible opportunities to minister to anyone who had a need.

We left the house at 8 a.m., and I was the first patient of the day. First, the techs did lab work to check my WBC count. Then, I met with the oncologist, who talked about previous test results (heart scan, bone density tests, and blood tests), time of recovery from this treatment (six to eight weeks to begin returning to normal energy level), and follow-up surgery and treatment. He is very thorough, and I am grateful. Then, I went to the treatment room to begin chemotherapy.

For the first time, they had problems getting my port to work, but they obviously knew what to do, so I prayed that things would go smoothly. It was not a day for complications — I had a sense of peace that the Lord was in control.

One of the chemicals I receive is known for attacking the heart. Before I am given that treatment, they normally give me another chemical first that is a "blocker." After I received the blocker, the other drug is infused very quickly so that the chemo drug attacks the blocker rather than my heart muscles.

However, yesterday, the blocker was not available anywhere in Texas. The oncologist gave me two choices. One was to wait another week or two for treatment in hope that the blocker would become available. We had no guarantees that the drug would be available anytime soon. The other choice was for me to have treatment yesterday as planned, but for them to give me the chemical very slowly. That was the doctor's recommendation, and that is what I did. The idea of postponing treatment was not appealing to me; I was ready. As a result, chemotherapy infusions began at 10 a.m. and finished at 5 p.m. I am *so* grateful that I did not have to do this for every treatment. It took almost five hours to administer the one chemotherapy drug, but I was very thankful for the precautions they took in infusing the drug as slowly as possible.

My new friend Colleen also had chemotherapy yesterday. She did not find out until before treatment that it was her last one. We celebrated with great joy! She brought me flowers and a card to celebrate my last day. Then, late in the afternoon, all of the precious people who work at the office and who have helped us through our treatment threw confetti at us, hugged us, blessed us, and gave us "completion certificates"! They had all written personal notes on the certificates. How special to have them celebrating with us and for us to get to celebrate together!

Carie and her children brought lunch and spent several hours with me, which allowed Charlie to leave the hospital to come home. He returned at 5 p.m. to take me home.

After Carie and the children left, I talked to a lady whom I have seen before. I asked how she was doing, and she said things were not going well. Her chemotherapy managed to accomplish only 50 percent of what it needed to do. She would go through chemotherapy again, but the oncologist is not optimistic that the next round of treatments will complete the work. She has had cancer for six years but still has things she wants to be part of, like the birth of her first grandchild this fall. She is mostly concerned about her 22-year-old son, who is not walking with the Lord. And she is struggling with dying and leaving her husband alone. I prayed for her, and she cried and said I was actually the second person who had prayed for her that day. My heart aches for her and so many others whom I have met who are dealing with life and death issues. Some know the Lord and others do not, and I pray that God will work in their lives and meet their needs.

Charlie and I stopped for a bite of dinner on the way home, and as he prayed over our meal, I began to cry. It dawned on me that I will not have to do this again! The gratitude overflowed my heart. I will walk through each day, rejoicing in the series of "lasts" that are ahead. I can do this in His strength and mercy, which have been the sustaining elements all along. What precious assurance that He is always with us and will not leave us, now or ever! That is worth celebrating.

❧ GUEST

It is interesting to me how this journey with you has given us a view into your life as well as the lives of others you've mentioned who are on the same path. These are people and situations we would not have known about had we not met them through you.

The details you give about treatments (your layman's explanations works well for me, as I have no background in medicine) take the mystery out of chemotherapy and bring light into an otherwise obscure view of the treatment. Understanding is one of the things that dispels fear. You have brought a measure of understanding about this process that will help others who may have to take that path. Now, it won't seem so scary to them.

How faithful is our Father and the Lord Jesus and the Holy Spirit! I rejoice that you got to the finish line.

May these next days and weeks hold precious moments with our Lord who calls us to "Come up higher!" That is the message He spoke to me this week as I have been claiming the intimacy that exists between us, though I do not always recognize it when I feel unworthy, confused, or doubtful. He speaks those words as His message to me when I find my mind in places of despair or doubt.

So my resolve is not to remain there; I say to myself, "Come up higher!" as David spoke to his soul in Psalm 42:5:

Why are you downcast, O my soul?
Why so disturbed within me?
Put your hope in God, for I will yet praise him,
my Savior and my God.

With love and prayers and thanksgiving,

Dianna

Monday, July 28 — Accepting Sufficient Grace, One Day at a Time

During the night when I could not sleep, I thought about when the children of Israel were wandering in the wilderness and God provided food for them called "manna." It fell fresh from heaven daily, and they were to gather only what they needed for that day. The day before the Sabbath, they gather two days' worth so they could rest on the Sabbath. If they gathered more manna any other time, it would spoil (Exodus 16:2–5, 12–35).

What does this have to do with anything? I guess I thought that as I came to the last round of chemotherapy and had to walk through the side effects for the last time, it would be easier because I would have the assurance that I would not have to go through it again. And I have rejoiced, and with many tears, at some of the "lasts" I have gone through. But that has not made it easier. I have found my patience getting thinner, and I want this to be over *now*.

What is the lesson? God's grace is only sufficient for the present moment. It is not something I can store up several days at a time. I cannot walk today in yesterday's grace. The patience I had three weeks ago is not sufficient for now. I have a greater demand for more strength and more endurance this week. *Grace cannot be stored like groceries in the freezer. It has to be fresh, like the manna.*

Each step of this process has been different, and I have been different. Though the side effects are similar, I am a different person today than I was three weeks ago. My perspective and endurance are different. Even when I walk through similar situations, they are never quite the same. And it takes a fresh measure of God's grace for each step.

Charlie told me about a Greek word, *poikilos*, which is like the color spectrums of the rainbow and is used for the English words "varied," "manifold," and "diverse." This word describes grace, which is not a one-size-fits-all commodity, but is unique and specific for each person and each situation.[30]

James 1:2–4 (NKJV) says, "My brethren, count it all joy when you fall into various (*poikilos*) trials, knowing that the testing of your faith produces patience. But let patience have *its* perfect work, that you may be perfect and complete, lacking nothing." Each "various" trial has specific grace to see us through that trial. Another version says, "But let endurance and steadfastness and patience have full play and do a thorough work, so that you may be [people] perfectly and fully developed [with no defects], lacking in nothing" (James 1:4 AMP).

Many people have said, "I could not go through what you are experiencing." But God gives us specific grace for our own particular lives and situations. You have grace for what you must face and I have grace for what I am going through. God's grace is sufficient for each of us. Grace is God's gift. We cannot earn it. But His Spirit gives it to us so we can walk obediently with Him. It comes, not in the "jumbo package" to last for months at a time, but moment by moment as we seek Him for the ability to walk through the next step of a challenge.

I *do* want this time of testing to have its *full* work in me, which means I must not wish any of it away or try to shortcut the process. I must keep pressing into the Lord each moment to receive all He has for this specific part of the journey.

Weariness and pain point me in the direction of giving up, but the end is in view. I don't want to give up and then find myself "incomplete" or "lacking." Giving up is too costly. So, today, I am seeking the Lord for His grace, His blessings and strength, and I am choosing joy and thanksgiving. Some days, the choice is more difficult than other days. And by the precious gift of God's amazing grace for this day, I am able to choose His will, His joy, and the patience that comes from His Holy Spirit.

❧ GUEST

Mom,

You've been running uphill in the race, and God is bringing you to a plateau, where you will run on even ground so you can recover. Still, as you run, you will require His strength to move on, so we will continue to cheer for you and pray for your strength, running alongside of you as we all head for the Prize.

I am so proud of you: of your humility, of your weakness, and your willingness to throw up your hands and say, "I need more of You *today*, God." If this were the only legacy you leave to Christie and me and to our children, you would have taught us all so much through this, but I continue to be stunned by the extension of His hand through you in this experience.

Love,
Carie

❧ GUEST

What a plan God has that each person's situation should be their platform for testimony, every testimony being important to the whole Body. Because suffering is so prevalent, many could not receive your testimony except that it comes out of suffering. Those who are perceived as having it easy would not have the power and penetration in their words like the words that come from another who is hurting, too. . . .

Trusting, with love,
Dianna

❧ GUEST

Praise God for His faithfulness and for your love and encouragement and truth of the promise that endurance, by *His* grace, will have its full and complete results. Your middle-of-the-night meditation could not have been more timely for me. I have been struggling with the same feelings that you described (thinking I was alone) and struggling to cling to and rest in His promise of grace. Oh the joy of fellowship, what a gift from our Shepherd King. Glory to God.

Love,
Colleen

Hooray for the last treatment!!! Hooray for your ability to know that you will not rebound overnight but to pray that the last treatment will prepare your body for the healing and to have the patience to let the warriors in your body remove all traces of cancer.

I'm drawn to the movie "Chariots of Fire" from the early '80s. One of the runners, a Christian, would not run on Sunday, believing that would violate God's commandments. A teammate took his place and let him run on another day of the week. The Christian runner was reading a Scripture in church on that Sunday — Isaiah 40:31 (KJV): "But they that wait upon the Lord shall renew their strength; they shall mount up with wings as eagles; they shall run, and not be weary; and they shall walk, and not faint." If you look back at verse 29, it says that He gives strength to the weary and increases the power of the weak.

God bless you as you renew your strength so you can soar with the eagles and share your strength with those of us who can learn from your journey these past few months.

Prayers and Hugs,
Debarah

Thursday, July 31 —
Reaching the Finish Line and a New Beginning

Yesterday, I went to the oncologist's office for blood tests. I was told that my WBC count was "acceptably low," to which I responded that I would rather be "acceptably" anything than "unacceptably" something! The results of the tests meant that I am not on antibiotics and my energy level has not completely bottomed out, as it did last month.

Last night, for the first time in months, I slept soundly, without getting up and without any medication! When I woke up this morning, I felt a "shift" occurring in my spirit and I tuned my ears to hear what the Spirit was saying. I could hardly concentrate on what I was hearing because I was overcome with joy.

The Lord began to give me insight as He put some pieces together. For several days, I have had some unusual thoughts. I thought back to many years ago, when I was pregnant for the first time and how I loved being pregnant—so much that I was concerned that I would miss being pregnant. If you have ever had a baby, you understand that once that baby arrives, no one has time to miss being pregnant!

Another thought going through my mind was that "Most experiences in life are not an 'end' but a door that leads to the next phase." I wrote that down early this week. It sounded logical but I did not understand what God was saying to me until this morning.

I have been running hard toward the "finish line" for weeks. However, the shift that came this morning was a change in perspective as the Lord said, *"It is not a 'finish line' you are running toward, but a 'starting line!'* This is not 'an end' but a door to walk through to the future. It is time for a new beginning."

Those nine months of carrying that baby were not simply for "being pregnant." That pregnancy was the means to a new life that was birthed as a result of the months of stretching and growing. In a similar way, the months of surgery, recovery, chemotherapy, and more recovery have not been only to heal and build endurance but also to point toward a fresh start in life with new perspective and purpose.

Things happen in life that can give us the feeling of finality, and many times it is the end of a lifestyle—life as we knew it. When this happens, it is impossible to even think of moving forward, and I personally believe God must change our perspective so we can move on. But because we are still alive, is it not "the end," and we still have purpose, destiny, and a work to accomplish. God's plans are *always* for "a future and a hope" (Jeremiah 29:11 NASB).

Our lives are not simply single events connected by time. Each circumstance is intended to be equipping for the next phase of life. As we cooperate with God and trust Him to work on our behalf, every situation becomes the means and the preparation for the future.

Throughout the Scriptures, the number eight traditionally means "new beginnings." At the beginning of this year, almost everything I read said it was to be a year of "new beginnings." That sounded wonderful and I had eager anticipation for what the coming year would bring. But when I was diagnosed with cancer in early January, the excitement about a "new beginning" was replaced with ideas of survival, healing, endurance, and living and coping one day, one event, one doctor's appointment, one treatment at a time.

This morning, when the Lord began speaking, He reminded me that this *is* a year of new beginnings. I have said I will never be the same again. I am sure there is more preparation yet ahead as I continue to recover and regain strength and health. But, today my focus is on the "starting line" and on God's plans for my future.

You most likely have been through difficult times. Often our desire is that those times end and end quickly. But when we get through the "valley of the shadow of death," we must get new, refocused lenses. We need to ask God what it is that He has for us in the days to come. Ask Him to use the past — the good things as well as the pain — to touch lives and bring others closer to Him. Ask Him to use all events of your life for your good (Romans 8:28) and for His glory. He *still* has a plan for our lives, and it is *still* a good plan.

I pray that you are walking today, as I am, with hope for your future and with a heart that anticipates a fresh beginning. That hope should be daily, knowing that His mercies, His compassions, are new every morning (Lamentations 3:22-23). God can use each of us in amazing ways and even change our perspective of the past and of the future. *May we run together with joy and endurance toward the greatest "starting line" of all, the one that will take us into an eternity with our Bridegroom and King, Jesus.*

⚜ GUEST

It is hard to believe sometimes that God can use some of the bad things that have happened in our lives for good (Romans 8:28), yet I remember that it was in praising God during the bad things in my life that I got free . . ..

Thanks for the love,
Darleen

Thursday, August 7 — Seeking New Direction

I am grateful that only two weeks after chemotherapy, the side effects are going away more quickly than I expected. Many of you have prayed for that, and I thank you. I am through the most painful part of the process and have not been nauseated for several days. That is a blessing. For months, water has tasted like chemicals, and most food has had little taste at all. But in the past two or three days, food and water have actually begun to taste like they are supposed to taste.

Fatigue is the main issue I am dealing with, though I have more energy than I have had. I am sleeping at night, which is another answer to prayer. On Monday, I will begin exercising at the local fitness center. Also, Charlie and I are getting ready to go on a vacation. I had thought the purpose was so I could get some rest and recuperation. However, as the Lord is speaking to me about running for the "starting line" rather than the finish line, I know that on our vacation I am to spend time seeking Him for new vision and direction for the future.

Proverbs 29:18 (KJV) says, "Where there is no vision, the people perish." It would be senseless for me to start a journey without a road map. I have heard it said, "If you don't know where you are going in life, any road will get you there." How do I know that I am on the right road, headed in the right direction, unless I have guidance?

When I taught in a Christian school many years ago, one senior student said, "If you aim high, you will land somewhere." It sounded interesting and even impressed the other students, but had nothing to do with hitting the target! I want to accomplish more than just some "good things" in life. I want to do everything God wants me to do (Ephesians 2:10) and become all I can be in Christ. That will take perseverance and persistence and will not happen automatically.

Many times in Scripture, as God's children, we are exhorted to "come," "seek," "press in," "draw near," "call," or "ask." As we pursue God, He delights in doing much more than we ask Him to do (Ephesians 3:20), and He loves to give us blessings and gifts that are beneficial to our lives (Luke 11:9–13; James 1:17).

My goals for my spiritual life have not always been specific. For example, I've wanted "to be a good Christian." I'm not even sure I could define what a "good Christian" is. Most often, a "good Christian" is described by "works" rather than character. Only God can determine what is "good." He looks at our hearts as well as our works. He alone knows if we are doing things out of Godly and unselfish motives and attitudes.

Sometimes my goals have been so vague or so big that I couldn't see any progress. "God, I want to save the world!" First of all, I can't "save" anyone, and I personally don't have the faith that I can impact the entire world. I *can* pray for and impact the lives of my family. I can impact my neighbors' lives (and we've prayed for several of our neighbors). And I believe that I can encourage many of the Japanese Christians when we go to Japan to minister. That is part of God's calling on Charlie's and my lives. But to touch the entire world? That is not for one person to do but takes each of us doing our part!

Other goals I've had were so small or shallow that they took no faith at all and were things I could accomplish in my own strength.

I am going to set aside the week of vacation to seek the Lord for *His* fresh vision for my life. I trust Him to show me the part of the road map that I need to move forward.

My desire and focus at present is for new direction. That may not mean for me to make a 180° turn but may simply be a *fresh* confirmation that the ministries I'm involved with are exactly what I am to be doing. A "new beginning" probably doesn't always mean to stop what I am doing and start a new project, but it may mean that I get renewed motivation. Or it may involve an enlargement of what I have been doing that will require increased faith. I don't know what the "new direction" will be, but I am looking forward to spending concentrated time seeking God for His guidance.

I return to the doctor next week to talk about the follow-up treatment. I have many questions for him before I begin taking long-term medication. Charlie and I are praying for wisdom.

❧ GUEST

I heard the voice of a seasoned woman of God in your journal—not the only time. Much of my adult life, I have tended to rush from Plan A to Plan B, feeling behind before I even got started. More recently, I have realized the importance of being still and listening, not just in between phases but during each step. And that is what I heard you say.

Shedding old tendencies is not just a matter of will but also a matter of action, intentionally stepping into the new and away from the old when, by habit, my old default is in place. I can be so frustrated in working on the book I am writing. It's overwhelming! I want to cry (sometimes I do). I want someone else to do it. But the Lord is quietly urging me to "Come up higher." He urges me to listen to His direction, and to know that He will bring me through this: I can either do it in His peace or through my frustration. It takes perseverance, but learning to let Him lead when I think I have to do it myself is what I am working on.

I appreciate your testimonies, one after another, and so appreciate the way you have allowed the Lord to touch other people's lives as you go through this process, like the score is not as important in the outcome as the way we got it. "It is how you play the game that counts."

May the Holy Spirit continue to pour into you wisdom and revelation (Ephesians 1:17) as you seek His will each step.

With love and prayers,
Dianna

Wednesday, August 13 — Beginning to Rebuild

Three weeks after my last treatment, I am grateful to say that the past week has been fairly normal with no pain or nausea, though I am tired. I began working out at the fitness center and believe that will help my energy level. Reality is setting in: I am finished with chemotherapy. Yeah!

Tomorrow, I have an appointment for lab work and to meet with the oncologist. But I will *not* proceed to the infusion room for treatment with chemicals and will *not* have another painful WBC booster shot. I do *not* have to go through the three-week process again. Ah, the reality! It is time to celebrate!

I have questions about the follow-up treatment after reading about the medications, so I will ask those questions of the oncologist tomorrow. Charlie and I are still praying for wisdom concerning what is next. I will have minor surgery to remove the port.

As I am watching the summer Olympics, I have realized that after the race is over, the long-distance runners and swimmers don't just stop running or swimming. They have to gradually cool down and stretch out their bodies. Many of them did not go to the Olympics to run or swim only one race, but after one race, they immediately prepare for another. They must continue to follow their disciplined routine. Discipline must be a lifestyle.

I suspect I still have much "stretching" to do, as well as the rebuilding of my daily routine and redefining what "normal life" means. The process of rebuilding will be a step-by-step process and will probably involve some unknowns. I cannot return to life as it was. Along with the exercising, I am beginning to learn more about nutrition and am "juicing" again to rebuild my strength and help clean out the chemicals that have been put into my body during the past eight months.

Please pray that Charlie and I will have wisdom as we talk with the oncologist tomorrow. Charlie and I need God's wisdom to know what questions to ask and to understand the answers.

Thank you again for your continued encouragement and prayers.

Friday, August 15 — Going with Compassion to Those in Need

Yesterday, I had blood tests and met with the oncologist. He said my blood count is back to normal and I can schedule the last minor surgery. I will have another heart scan in two weeks to ensure the last chemotherapy didn't negatively affect my heart muscles. The doctor explained the follow-up plan to my satisfaction and in such a way that I could understand what is involved and why I should have this particular treatment. He pronounced me "cancer free" and said that all future treatment is to keep the breast cancer from returning to another part of the body. I did not realize that was a possibility.

Charlie and I are at peace, and I will begin the new daily medication in two weeks. I will also have infusions every six months to help rebuild my bones and to prevent osteoporosis. The follow-up treatment has been approved by our insurance company, which is a praise. The medication and infusions he recommended are both proven to help protect women from cancer recurrence.

My main prayer request at this point is that I will not have the possible side effects to these two medications. They are numerous and can be far less than desirable. This is another step of faith in trusting that the Lord is guiding and directing my life.

In the meantime, I am attempting to be disciplined about going to the fitness center. I am slowly beginning, as I mainly use the treadmill. I know the exercise is building my heart and my leg and hip muscles. They are weak because I have not exercised over the past year or so. I am also hoping the exercise will help to burn off some of the weight I have gained while going through chemotherapy. I have found weight gain to be one of the most discouraging side effects for many people going through treatment.

In some ways, I find exercising at the fitness center to be very unsatisfying. I walk, jog, and even climb hills on the treadmill, but I don't get anywhere. I am working my muscles, but I stay in one place. It seems that much of my spiritual life has been like that. I go to church and exercise my spiritual muscles through studying the Word, worshiping, praising, and praying. However, so much of the Lord's direction involves the word "Go." It involves movement: purposeful direction and intentional motion. I once heard, "Two-thirds of 'God' is 'Go'!" Yet, often I seem to fall short in the "going" part of my spiritual life.

The Great Commission tells us to "Go into all the world and preach the Gospel" (Mark 16:15 HCSB). Other Scriptures also tells us to "Go":

- "As you go, preach, saying, 'The Kingdom of Heaven is at hand!' Heal the sick, cleanse the lepers, and cast out demons. Freely you received, so freely give" (Matthew 10:7–8 HNV).

- ". . . If a man has a hundred sheep, and one of them goes astray, does he not leave the ninety-nine and go to the mountains to seek the one that is straying?" (Matthew 18:12 NKJV).

- "If you want to be perfect, go, sell what you have and give to the poor, and you will have treasure in heaven; and come, follow Me" (Matthew 19:21 NKJV).

- "Go therefore and make disciples of all the nations, baptizing them in the name of the Father and of the Son and of the Holy Spirit, teaching them to observe all things that I have commanded you" (Matthew 28:19–20).

These are clear instructions to those who consider themselves to be followers of Christ. Yet, often, I find myself caught up in my own life and I forget about other people. I don't reach out but wait for others to come to me. I "stay" rather than "go." I don't pursue people who are lost and needy, and I sometimes even avoid them.

The past few months of visiting the hospital has changed my perspective, as I have talked with hurting people. As a result, my heart has cried out for God to give me opportunities to touch lives with the Gospel. I want to go after the "lost sheep." I want Him to send me to those who do not know Him and have no hope.

I know what hope is. I know what love, encouragement, and support are. And, at the same time, I am able to remember what "lostness" and "hopelessness" are like. I have hope and know the love and power of God because someone obeyed the go-and-tell part of the Gospel and shared it with me. I have freely received much from the Lord and want to share it with others. That means I need to get outside of the walls of the church and my home and touch the lives of those who will not "come" to hear the Gospel.

I have written before that I do not have to look far to find people who are walking through more difficult trials than I have faced. I talked to a lady at the oncologist's office yesterday who has lung cancer and has been through several rounds of chemotherapy. The disease in one lung is responding, but the disease in the other is not. As I talked with her, wanting to encourage her, she encouraged me. She wanted to know how I was doing and rejoiced that I was finished with chemotherapy.

It doesn't take much to "go," only a heart for people, a desire to share the goodness of the Lord, and a little boldness. And when I don't have the boldness, but do have compassion, God makes up the difference and helps me to reach out. I must also consciously value each person I meet — not as a waiter, an employee, or someone to serve me, but as a person created by God who has feelings, potential, and eternal destiny.

Wednesday evening, I heard a teaching on being "love deficient." Love for others is proven by compassion in our hearts. I heard again that I can be "spiritual" and do many good works, but if I don't have love, I am nothing and what I do is useless (1 Corinthians 13). I pray that God will continue to build love and compassion in my heart for others. I believe He gives us opportunities every day to be His ambassador to share Him with others. I want to recognize those opportunities and take advantage of them.

❧ GUEST

Your entry about "going" is one to which I relate so well. I *hated* my treadmill: facing the wall, exercising and yet seeing no progress except the 1 or 2 lbs each week that I'd lose. Over time, I saw my body shape change a little and that was encouraging, but to "go" and see the progress meant I also had to "wait" and "persevere." Those are not characteristics I strongly bear.

You have done a lot of waiting and persevering in the last year. You've had to sit during your infusions and recover, and yet God has used that time to grow you and has used you to bless and challenge others.

I love you and rejoice that you are *here* and not back in January. God has been faithful, even in the suffering, and He has saved you for the work He has in store. While every trip to Japan is precious, this next trip is a unique victory walk, for God may have saved you from cancer so you will "go" this time. How exciting!

Carie

GUEST

This week I shared vegetables from the garden with our neighbors and friends. I had the thought that it would be wonderful to give them to someone that really needs them, that maybe can't afford them. The other night, one friend was so glad to get the food as her paycheck was delayed, and they had nothing left in their bank account. And today, I shared some with the FedEx man, who has a large family.

Our thoughts were on the same page today. I told the Lord that I know He goes to the lost sheep, and we are willing and ready (RVs and all), but I asked Him if I ever got to the point that I couldn't physically "go" would He bring them as He brought the man that needed vegetables. (I have a Bible "doer" group at the nursing home now, and that is what we talked about last Wednesday. They want to "go" somewhere to find the lost sheep, and the lost sheep might be right there among them.)

Hope this is encouragement to you as you go forward. You minister to people at your check-ups, and everywhere God takes you! We praise Him for His wonderful works everywhere you "go."

With love and blessings to you and Charles and your family,

Thomas and Abigale

Thursday, August 21 — Pacing Myself and Prioritizing

Four weeks ago, I had my last chemotherapy treatment. I still have moments when it freshly dawns on me that I will not have more chemotherapy. I still have some eyebrows and eyelashes and all of my fingernails and toenails! I rejoice in the small things! I have lost a few pounds and believe that is mainly because the swelling in my legs and feet is going down — another praise.

When I was a child, early September represented a "fresh start" as a new school year began. That doesn't affect me as much now that I'm not in school and we don't have children at home, but as September approaches, I still think of all that comes with a new school year: new notebooks, crayons and pencils, clothes, and lunch box and a new teacher. I was always excited about the new opportunity. I feel like I am there once again.

Another issue God is impressing on my heart concerns pacing myself to protect my energy and my time. As we watched the women's marathon earlier in the Olympics, Charlie pointed out that the women set their watches before the race so they could pace themselves. As they came to check points along the way, they could see if they were putting out too much energy too early in the race, or if they were holding back and not running fast enough.

With my limited energy, I, too, must pace myself. Pacing starts with prioritizing what I need to do each day and concentrating my energy on those things. I often begin a job but get distracted and begin to do other things that are not necessary at that time.

At our house in the country, we always have much to do — projects to finish and new ones to begin. When I get distracted by all that needs to be done, I have problems sticking to the important task at hand. I don't always use my time wisely, so I run out of energy before I finish what I need to do.

I need discipline to do only those things that need to be done each day and then stop and rest. This is a big change for me. In the past, when I got diverted, I stayed up late at night, pushing myself to get everything done. I cannot do that now with my low energy level.

The Lord continues to speak to me from the book of Hebrews about rest. I am trying to obey and discipline myself to stop and rest. I am praying that God's fruit of self-control (Galatians 5:22-23) will grow strong in me.

As the summer comes to an end, may you have renewed strength and hope to begin the fall and head into the last few months of the year. May the Lord give you a fresh beginning each day.

Monday, September 8 — Learning to Rest, Again

I have not posted a journal in weeks, but it has been an amazing few weeks.

Charlie and I went on the most wonderful vacation we have ever experienced. We took a cruise up the inland pass of Alaska. By the time Charlie took his third nap on our first day at sea, he felt guilty. We spent most of our time on the ship either eating, roaming around the ship, or resting, sleeping, studying, reading in our room and looking at the beautiful scenery — the ocean, mountains, waterfalls, and glaciers. The magnificent scenery had a healing and restoring effect on us. We returned home rested.

The Lord talks much in the Scriptures about rest, which is primarily an inner condition. "Christ's 'rest' is not a 'rest' *from* work, but *in* work, 'not the rest of inactivity but of the harmonious working of all the faculties and affections — of will, heart, imagination, conscience — because each has found in God the ideal sphere for its satisfaction and development".[31] To me that says that the result of a restful life is *satisfaction*.

In our world today, it is difficult to find peaceful, quiet places. To align our will, heart, imagination, and conscience with God, we must take time to listen to Him. That requires finding a place away from the noises of the world so we can tune into His voice.

I have shared that Charlie and I have wonderful "quiet" in the country where we live, and I love it. I can easily hear God's voice as I sit on the back deck and look at the pasture and the pond or listen to the sounds of the birds chirping and the creek running. But man-induced sounds tend to compete with the voice of the Lord, and the noise of the world does not draw me into a place of rest and peace. The stress of traffic and the busy rush of people in the big city compete with God's rest.

Rest is something we discover and enter into and then take with us. I must have my heart in a resting position before I head to the hospital, so I can carry the peace of God in my heart to hurting people who are often stressed and worried.

As we began the cruise, I quickly became aware of how the last nine months have drained Charlie's energy. He began to rest immediately, when normally it takes him time to shift gears from his busy life and begin to rest. During this year, Charlie carried the load of responsibility. I originally thought the vacation was for my benefit but quickly recognized that it was for his also. I am grateful for the lavish provision of this trip. It brought restoration and satisfaction to our minds, bodies, and souls.

Monday, September 15 — Welcoming God's Infusion

I am learning to release my expectations. I expected that by this time, my physical strength would be normal. I am still experiencing side effects from treatments, and I realize the journey is not over. I don't know when or if it will ever end. Some of the physical side effects did not begin to show up until the past few weeks. I become tired quickly and my capacity for activity is limited. I have to use wisdom and caution about moving back into ministry and a fast-paced life.

Also, I still have times of emotional reaction. Recently I walked into the guest bedroom and bathroom where I spent much time during the past six months, and the smells of those rooms reminded me of chemotherapy and almost made me sick. Recently, I was reading my daily schedules of the past few months, and when I came to the sentence "Today is chemotherapy session . . . ," I began to weep. I still don't know why, but I do realize that I experienced physical as well as emotional impacts of the treatments. I suspect this is probably true of any crisis.

I suspect that I will never return to "normal life." Too much has changed. I wonder why we think we can go back in life when life should be forward motion with progress and change. And, as the last eight months have caused me to learn to persevere, I also realize that perseverance must become a *lifestyle*, not just a *season of life*.

In recent weeks, the word "infusion" has been difficult if not impossible for me to consider. When I think about returning to the lab for another infusion, I find myself in tears. And, as before, as I read the lists of possible side effects of the medications, I become overwhelmed and am unsure if I can go through with it. I have watched a dear friend whose maintenance treatment has been more difficult and challenging than the chemotherapy. So, again, I am going to the Lord with my resistance, fears, and dread. God continues to work deeper in my heart in those areas.

Yesterday, I drove alone to church. We normally use the hour of driving time to worship. But as I was driving, the Lord began to speak to me, saying, "Be still, and know that I am God" (Psalm 46:10). With an awe of the Lord strongly welling up inside me, I turned the music off and tuned my heart to hear His voice. He began talking about His infusion into my life, telling me about all He is pouring into me. I was overwhelmed because His words brought redemption to the word "infusion" and immediately removed the dread that had been attached to that word.

As soon as I got home, I checked the dictionary. Webster[32] defines *infuse* (the root of *infusion*), which is from the term "to pour in" and means "to instill a principle or quality in; introduce; inspire; to steep in water or other fluid without boiling for extracting useful qualities. *To infuse implies a pouring in of something that gives new life or significance.*" In the physical, it is the "introduction of a solution into a vein." Yet, in the spiritual, it is also an introduction, an impartation of new things into my life. That has truly happened this year, as I have experienced God's presence in new ways, developed a new level of compassion, grown in faith and trust, and experienced new freedom in areas where I previously experienced fear.

The physical introduction of a solution into my veins has had the effect of giving new and healthy life. It has also removed things (cancer cells) in my system that bring death. In the spiritual realm, the same is true. The Lord has infused life-giving truths into my heart and mind that have removed many fears, discouragement, unhealthy attitudes, and lies of the enemy.

Why is this important? It is vital that *nothing be allowed to steal my joy, my destiny, or my purpose in life.* I am willing to fight for those things. When even an ungodly thought or word of fear, doubt, or accusation ("fiery darts of the evil one" Ephesians 6:16 ASV) strikes at my heart, I must deal with it immediately or, like cancer, it begins to eat up my soul and steal life from me.

God continues to show me the truth in His Scripture that He can use any situation for the good of those who love Him (Romans 8:28). Many times, I remind Him that I know He will use this situation for my good because He promised and He does not ever go back on His promises. He is God of the impossible (Matthew 19:26; Mark 10:27).

So, I will move forward, trusting in God's character shown in John 2:1–11 and through Jesus's first miracle of turning water into wine: *God truly saves the best for last.* He can turn our mourning into joy, our fears into confidence, and our dread into hope, even as He turned death into resurrected life. Together, let us look forward with expectation to God's character being revealed in a deeper way in and through our lives. He is Faithful and gives good gifts to His children. And that is worth celebrating!

❦ GUEST

Lately, I've been rereading my favorite passages of Scripture from *The Message* and I remembered the term *steep*. So I looked it up again. I pass this to you as encouragement.

"Steep your life in God-reality, God-initiative, God-provisions. Don't worry about missing out. You'll find all your everyday human concerns will be met" (Matthew 6:33 MSG).

Isn't that great! God is good—all the time!!

Choose joy, my friend,
Lissa

❦ GUEST

I understand the association between sights and smells and thoughts of chemo. I had moments like that as well. Get a nice, new air freshener to put in those rooms. Create a new association.

I know how hard it is to not really be finished. People expect things of you and you expect things of yourself. But it sounds like God is reminding you to take the time to heal, both physically and emotionally. There will always be reminders that trigger some tears. Just the other day, I was reading back through a private journal I wrote during the days after my diagnosis and leading up to my surgery and I started crying as I relived all those emotions.

Thank you for your inspiring words and for allowing God to work through you, using your life crisis to impart such wisdom to so many.

Love,
Susan

What determines the choices we make each day? How do we decide what to do, what not to do, and how to use our time? How do we determine what we are going to accomplish? I have been asking myself these questions. My energy level and strength are beginning to increase, and I am eager to see progress in some important areas of my life. Yet, I struggle with using my time wisely.

A friend once told me that it is almost impossible to *find time* to do the important things in life. Instead, we must *make time* for them. If we don't *make time*, the important things will not happen. This principle has become a challenge to me. I have not accomplished many things, simply because I did not make time to do them. Instead, I often respond to that which is urgent at the moment, rather than persevering with what is most important.

By the time I became a Christian, my destiny seemed fixed. I was a military wife who frequently packed, moved, unpacked, and reestablished our household. I raised our children, fixed meals, kept house, worked at church, and sometimes worked outside of the home. We would live somewhere for one to four years. About the time we were settled, Charlie would get orders, and the process would start again.

When I worked full-time, my structure was established. I would work all day, and I had little energy when I got home from work. The weekends were for cleaning, catching up, and going to church, and if there was time and energy left over, we would go to a movie or spend time with friends. I didn't think much about vision or calling but did what the day demanded.

During the past nine months, we've lost the structure of a "regular schedule." My strength and energy have dictated what I could do. I have struggled with lack of accomplishment. Charlie has been very faithful to remind me that rest was (and still is) necessary for my healing. Some days, when survival was the goal, anything I did beyond that was success, even if it was only to fix a meal or do a load of laundry.

When Charlie and I were on vacation, I spent time seeking the Lord's plan for my future. I prayed for fresh vision. In the past, much of my vision has been intertwined with Charlie's. But the Lord has spoken that we are in a new season, and new vision is necessary. It is a different experience for me to seek fresh vision for my individual life because Charlie and I have ministered together for many years.

Perhaps this is not unique to me. Many times, I meet women whose lives are so intertwined with their husbands' or their children's activities that they feel like their purpose is limited or nonexistent apart from their families. But God, in His infinite wisdom, created us individually, called us as individuals, and fashioned within each of us gifts and abilities for the destiny He designed us for.

Now, as I face the future, I don't have the built-in structure of work, and my children are grown. I need guidelines for how to spend my time and energy.

I have never been especially good at goal setting. My idea of goals has been to be a better wife, mother, or Christian. As you can probably guess, my experience with goal setting has been very unsatisfactory. I only recently found out that the reason for that was because my goals were not measurable! "Better" is relative and does not have an attainable measurement. (See entry for August 7—"Seeking New Direction.")

Charlie has always had a one, five, and ten-year plan. He is helping me set measurable goals. I still want to be better at the things I do, but am taking a different approach by doing some specific planning.

Why is this important? This past year, I have come to a deeper realization of the value of life. I don't want to spend my time doing meaningless tasks or simply responding to the urgency of the moment. But, *desire is not enough*. Without a specific plan followed by action, I can easily drift back to the same old patterns of life.

He had wonderful plans for my life even before I was born (Psalm 139:16) and I want to know what they are. It takes determination to listen to Him, and not listen to what even well-meaning people may want or think. I must learn to say "no" to the many things that pull at my life and some that even tug at my heart but that do not align with His best plans for me.

Many of you have prayed that I would have "life." I now see that life is far more than health. It includes fulfilling my destiny.

Thank you for your prayers and support. May the Lord pour His *life* and purpose into you in a fresh way today. I pray for those of you who are younger, that you will discover these principles for your life before you reach my age—and especially for you who have walked through crises and found it difficult to "begin again." I pray that the God who created you with a purpose and plan will draw you near and whisper into your heart that you are valuable to Him. May you never doubt that He still has things for you to do that will impact the Kingdom of God.

GUEST

I never really considered "pro-life" to be anything other than antiabortion. After watching you choose to fight cancer, struggle through chemotherapy, and emerge even more aware of the value of life — each moment of each day — I have realized that "pro-life" is so much more: it's recognizing that this moment is valuable and analyzing how we use it to glorify God.

Thank you for sharing this and sharing with me on the phone today. I love being your daughter! (I get special access!)

Carie

GUEST

Thank you for this update that speaks so well about things in my own heart. Personal responsibility in responding to God with my own life, not subjectively, but with a fuller awareness of God's destiny and the fact that time is limited, has become a stronger and clearer focus recently. Like you, I want others to see that! Life is *so not ordinary* in the Kingdom of Heaven. . . .

As I watch some outspoken Christian women in the political public eye, whom I believe to be living on the cutting edge of God's destiny, I see that, like a surfer riding a wave, their widespread impact looks adventuresome and fun, but it also involves risks, humanly speaking, and costs. . . . Yet, God actually wants to change the world through us. . . . God does not expect the government to do what He has called the Church to do! Seeking first the Kingdom of God and His righteousness means so much more than being a faithful church goer!

God is speaking to me about overcoming fears that have gone unnoticed but that have restricted me from loving God with all my heart and strength! I, too, seek to hear His voice, His call, and be ready to carry it out completely, today. May we walk in His grace and His truth and so fulfill our Kingdom purposes.

Love and Kingdom blessings to you,

Dianna

Wednesday, October 1 — Keeping My Eyes on the Lord

In the past nine months, the Lord has repeatedly told me that I must keep my eyes on Him and not on my circumstances. That is not always easy but is how I endured even the most painful days.

How do we keep our eyes on Him when we as humans cannot "see" God with our physical eyes? Focusing on Him means that our heart — our mind, will, and emotions — is stirring with God's Word. The Scriptures are filled with revelation of His character and with His promises to us. As we study and meditate on His Word, not only does it keep our thoughts off the worries and possibilities of our situations, but we begin to have His perspective and our faith in Him grows stronger. When Jesus becomes our Lord, He wants to be Lord of everything in our lives all of the time. He is not a "part-time" God. He cares about everything we face and is able to handle the small things as well as the large things in our lives. My life bears witness that He keeps His promises.

I can teach you how to *not* do just about anything. It is a good thing that I am able to learn from my mistakes! And yesterday I realized once again that living by my own expectations and plans is not how to keep my focus on the Lord.

I made an appointment five weeks ago with the surgeon to have my chemotherapy port removed, which is a minor surgical procedure. I was looking forward to having this behind me. However, when I got to the surgeon's office, the doctor had no idea that my appointment was to remove my port, so I only had a short physical exam and now must return later to have the port removed. When the situation was not what I had expected, I became disappointed and frustrated (which I have been told is a nice word for "angry.") I had to work through the situation, forgive the person who miscommunicated, and walk in the peace that comes from trusting that the Lord guides my steps (Psalm 37:23).

I have asked myself how I will handle extreme situations if I can't even keep my focus on the Lord in the smaller matters of life, like a change in schedule due to someone's mistake. I cannot control what happens in my life, in our nation, or in the world. But I am responsible for controlling my attitudes and responses. My deepest desire is for Him to be glorified in every attitude, word, action, and reaction of my life.

God tells us that at all times we are to have hope in Him. Hope is "favorable and confident expectation" and "has to do with the unseen and the future".[33] Putting my hope in His plans differs from establishing my own expectations.

Many times in the Psalms, King David wrote about the trials he was going through as his enemies pursued him. Yet, even in the midst of those trials, he put his hope in the Lord (e.g., Psalm 42:10–11; 53:5; 71:5, 14.) I especially love Psalm 146, which tells us to put our hope in the Lord and then lists numerous reasons why that is possible.

Jeremiah the prophet said,

> Thus says the Lord, "Cursed is the man who trusts in man and makes flesh his strength, whose heart departs from the Lord. . . . Blessed *is* the man who trusts in the Lord, and whose hope is the Lord. For he shall be like a tree planted by the waters, which spreads out its roots by the river, and will not fear when heat comes; but its leaf will be green, and will not be anxious in the year of drought, nor will cease from yielding fruit" (Jeremiah 17:5, 7–8 NKJV).

When I live by my own expectations, I am trusting in myself and my reasoning rather than in the all-knowing God. I prefer to live under the blessings of the Lord rather than the consequences of my own weak and imperfect understanding and abilities. The benefits of trusting Him are practical and pertinent to today. His promises *cannot* fail but are activated when we put our faith in Him and His Word.

In the same chapter, Jeremiah prays to the Lord, "You *are* my hope in the day of doom" (Jeremiah 17:17 NKJV). Later, Jeremiah says,

> *Through* the Lord's mercies we are not consumed, because His compassions fail not. *They are* new every morning; Great *is* Your faithfulness. "The Lord *is* my portion," says my soul, "Therefore I hope in Him!" The Lord *is* good to those who wait for Him, to the soul *who* seeks Him. It is good that *one* should hope and wait quietly for the salvation of the Lord (Lamentations 3:22-26 NKJV).

As I know and trust His amazing character of love, goodness, faithfulness, holiness and His awesome power, I will have confident expectation. As my journey progresses, the Lord daily reveals His trustworthiness to me.

Today, I had the first infusion that is part of the follow-up treatment. The infusion took longer than I expected. The oncologist also sent me for a sonogram to see if I had any blood clots in my legs that might be causing my feet to continue to swell. I do not have blood clots, and so far, I have experienced no side effects from the medication I received. Thank you for praying.

God continues to use the issues of my daily walk to restore my health, to clean out my heart and to conform me to His image. It is a good work He is doing!

Monday, October 6 — Experiencing Effects from My Follow-up Infusion

The infusion I had last week is supposed to strengthen my bones and prevent osteoporosis as well as a reoccurrence of cancer. However, the side effects include weakness and much pain in my bones. Walking has been difficult, and climbing stairs and standing has been a challenge. I am praying that this pain will decrease before we leave for Japan, where we walk many miles and stand for hours.

Your prayers make a difference. I know God has called us to Japan, so we are trusting Him to provide everything we need. As I keep my eyes on Him rather than on my weakness, I have faith. When I focus on myself, my faith weakens, and rightly so! He alone is to be the *object* as well as the *source* of our faith.

P.S. My hair is growing. Charlie calls me "fuzzy!" The growth *is* progress.

Tuesday, October 7 — Knowing God Is in Control

Do you believe that God does not make mistakes? He cares for His children, and the details of our lives are not hidden from Him. He is faithful (Deuteronomy 7:9; Revelation 19:11)!

Last week, I wrote that the surgeon did not remove my port on Tuesday, as I expected. Yesterday, I received a call from the surgeon's office and, because of complications with my paperwork, I was "lost in the system" and my referrals had expired. Therefore, I did not have insurance coverage last week. Had my port come out per *my* plans, we would have had to pay for the entire cost of the procedure! How I rejoice that I am never "lost" to

God. I attributed the situation to "inefficiency of man" and lack of communication. But God says even when I make plans, He guides my steps (Proverbs 16:9), . . . and I forgot that truth.

Even after 38 years as a Christian, I still don't always think with a "Kingdom mindset." Instead, I reason. Why do I not trust that God is still in control when things do not go according to my plans? God is committed to doing what is best for us. He knows all things (Ezekiel 11:5; Psalm 139:2). He knows the "what if's" (Matthew 11:21–24; 1 John 3:20). He knows all the details and has promised to provide for us according to His all-knowing ability (Philippians 4:19). God loves (Romans 8:31–32, 35) and cares about us, . . . even when we don't see it. He is all powerful (Psalm 62:11) and can control every situation. I continue to pray that He will make me flexible. I pray to have wisdom that allows me to see with His eyes, hear with His ears, feel with His heart, and live relying on Him rather than on my human understanding (Proverbs 3:5–6).

So after more than three hours on the phone, our insurance issues are resolved and we celebrate all that the Lord has done for us in the practical realms of our lives.

❧ GUEST

I had never read Corrie ten Boom's *The Hiding Place*[34], until last week. It is an amazing testimony and has really left an impression on me. Your journal entry today brought to mind something from the book that happened between Corrie and her sister, Betsie, while they were prisoners in a concentration camp in Germany. The room where they slept and the straw on which they slept were infested with fleas. Corrie was especially horrified and asked Betsie how they were ever going to be able to stand it. Betsie's answer was taken from Scripture, and she said they would get through it by thanking God in all circumstances. So together, they agreed that they were thankful to God that they had not been separated and that God had protected Corrie from being searched so she was able to smuggle in her Bible. Then, Betsie thanked God for the fleas, and Corrie went along with it, feeling sure that Betsie was wrong on that one. But, later they noticed that none of the guards ever entered the room and they couldn't understand why. This made it possible for them to read their Bible together and share the Gospel with 1400 other women in the back of the room.

Later, they found out that the guards didn't come in because of the fleas!

So, yes, your recent experience is another reminder that God is working out everything for our good and His glory. Thanks for sharing!

Love,
Cathy

Monday, October 13 — Being Inoculated against God

This afternoon, Charlie and I each received a flu shot. I needed a flu shot because my immune system is still low. As the doctor explained, the inoculation is made of the flu cells and receiving a small dose keeps us from getting the full-blown flu. On the way home, I began to think of how our spiritual lives are often like that flu shot. The flu shot is a good thing, but the same principle can also work against us. When we allow ourselves a bit of sin, that small amount keeps us from receiving the full infilling of the Holy Spirit. When we justify our sin, our consciences become deadened, or inoculated, to the convicting power of the Holy Spirit.

The apostle John wrote,

> If we say that we have no sin, we deceive ourselves, and the truth is not in us. If we confess our sins, He is faithful and just to forgive us *our* sins, and to cleanse us from all unrighteousness. If we say that we have not sinned, we make Him a liar, and His word is not in us (1 John 1:8-10 NKJV).

When we fall short of confession and repentance, we keep the sin in our lives. But through repentance, we are set free from sin. Repentance involves agreeing with God; confessing that we need Him to change us; and then receiving His power and grace which allow us to change.

The apostle Paul wrote, ". . . lay aside every weight, and the sin which so easily ensnares *us*, and let us run with endurance the race that is set before us, looking unto Jesus, the author and finisher of *our* faith . . ." (Hebrews 12:1-2 NKJV). The Scriptures tell us we are all sinners (Romans 3:23), so why don't we get rid of the sin? Why do we cling to it or excuse it?

I think of what I have gone through to get rid of cancer. It has not been fun. I don't want to ever have to go through it again. But it was worth all I went through to be cancer-free.

Then, I think of what Jesus went through on the cross to rid us of the spiritual cancer of sin. We have only to accept what He did for us and His Holy Spirit will enter our hearts and begin to clean out the sin in our lives. How amazing a healing is that! Why would we refuse such a life-changing gift? I pray that we will not inoculate ourselves against the Spirit of God, who wants to give us spiritual healing.

John also wrote, "Beloved, I pray that in all respects you may prosper and be in good health, just as your soul prospers" (3 John 1:2 NASB). I enjoy life and I desire good health. But I especially want to live with prosperity of my soul, which involves spiritual wholeness. That is possible because of God's great love. My physical healing has been only a part of His amazing blessings that flow from His Spirit of love. How great He is!

May we allow the power of His love to accomplish His good work within us and make us healthy and whole.

Wednesday, October 15 — Preparing to Travel

Charlie and I are prepared, and we fly out early tomorrow to Japan for ten days of ministry. We planned a shorter trip this time since my energy level is low. However, as our schedule has come together, we have only one free day, and that is the day after we arrive, which will allow us to get unpacked and begin to get over jet lag. We will minister at least once and sometimes twice each day. It would have been so easy to stay home and not go to Japan this fall, but God has something special for us to do on this trip, and we are excited.

One of our friends, a Japanese pastor, is praying for and seeing an increasing number of people healed. However, his wife was diagnosed with breast cancer about a year ago and the cancer has spread. She and I completed chemotherapy at the same time. Charlie and I will minister at this pastor's healing services two nights next week. We are praying for his wife to have complete healing.

Thank you to all who have committed to pray for us as we travel and minister. We believe this trip is going to be an exceptional blessing in our lives.

Tuesday, October 21 — Sharing My Testimony in Japan

We arrived safely in Japan and all is going well. We are very busy, and God is touching lives. He is using my testimony of all He has done in the past year to minister here. I had not expected that.

Thank you for your prayers for health and strength. Many of the people we have prayed for are sick with flu and colds. We are very tired after ministering, but we have had the strength to do what God has called us here to do. We are grateful.

Friday, October 24 — Glorifying God in Time of Crisis

This trip has been different for me in many ways. Often, when we get ready to travel to Japan, I sense an underlying and subtle sense of doubt with thoughts like, "This is so difficult. I hope God will give me the messages and anoint my teachings. Will our words impact lives?" This time, I recognized those feelings and thoughts as *unbelief*. In the past, I have ignored them and kept going. Before this trip, I stopped and dealt with them. There is a huge difference.

As we prepared for our trip and the doubt would arise, I would immediately confess it as sin — as contrary to God's plan — and then profess what I know to be true about God. The immediate result was that my doubt was replaced with joy, and I faced this trip with an anticipation that I've not had in the past.

The Lord continues to deal with me concerning living a Kingdom life and seeing things from His perspective rather than living with worldly vision and based on feelings.

In the middle of the night last Sunday, I began praying for the morning meeting, "God will you please anoint the message? Will you touch lives? Will you give me the right words to say?" In the middle of my "prayer," I heard the Lord say, "STOP!" I did, and I waited. Then He said, "Now, pray with faith!" And I began again,

> Lord, thank You that You have sent us here to deliver Your message. Thank You that You have prepared their hearts to receive Your Word, and Your Word does not return void. It accomplishes Your purposes as You have said (Isaiah 55:11). I expect fruitfulness to be the result of our ministry time in Japan. And I thank You for the

privilege of being chosen to come here and speak forth
Your truth and Your goodness to these precious people.
In Jesus' name, I thank and praise You.

WOW! What a work that prayer did in my heart. It affirmed who God is, what He wants, and what He has called us to do. *Praying truth, with faith focused on God and His plans, can change the atmosphere.* It shut the door to the enemy as it filled me with confident expectation rather than questioning, doubting, begging, or wondering.

Last night, I spoke at a healing service of 40–50 people. On the way to Tokyo yesterday morning, the Lord gave me the message I was to share, "Glorifying Christ in Time of Crisis." I got excited. One of the Scriptures He gave me was in Daniel 3, about the three young men who were thrown in the fiery furnace because they would not do things the world's way. They would not bow down to the idol of the pagan king. When I reread the familiar Scripture, it touched my heart in a new and deep way. The three men said, "Our God can deliver us from the fire. But, if He does not, we will still serve Him" (paraphrase of Daniel 3:17–18). I felt that way last January, knowing that my God could instantly heal me of cancer, but if He did not, I knew that I would continue to serve Him, praise Him, and trust Him for His work in my life.

Several years ago, our daughter Carie gave me some special insight into this story. She reminded me that three men were thrown into the fire. But, when the king looked into the furnace, he saw *four* men, and even the pagan king recognized that the fourth man looked "like the Son of God" (Daniel 3:25 NKJV). Carie asked me, "How many men came out of the fire?" and I responded, "Three." She said, "Yes, Mom. Three came out, but *the Son of God stayed in the fire so He would be there with you and me when we are in the midst of fiery trials.*"

How many times does God say, "Fear not because I am with you"? His presence makes the difference.

My desire for my own life is to be like the three young men in the fiery furnace, who not only came out of the fire alive and not harmed but also did not smell like smoke. Only the ropes that were used to bind them were burned. God can use even the fiery experiences through which we walk to set us free from the bondages of sin which keep us from fully trusting God.

Our time here is going by quickly, and we come home in only four days. Thank you again for your prayers. They are making a difference. We do need increased strength as we finish these last few days.

Friday, October 31 — Changing Is Essential to Life

Charlie and I are home again; laundry is almost finished, suitcases are empty, we have shopped for groceries, and we have had our "Mexican-food fix" after all the good low-fat food we ate in Japan. Our bodies are still not quite on Texas time, but we are sleeping during the night and are gradually transitioning into routine Texas life again.

Transition is a good word for "change." Change describes the Christian life. Often we try to keep things the same, and when they begin to shift, we get nervous, feel insecure, and try to do what we can to get them back to the way things were before. We like to control our lives and we like our comfort zones. But we can't live in the past or go backwards. Going forward involves change.

I am grateful that God does not impose change simply for the sake of change but always for our benefit and according to His loving and divine plan. We should be constantly moving forward, progressing, and changing into the image of the character of God. God gives much practical direction as to how that process can come about and how we can become more like Him than like the world (e.g., Romans 13:14; Ephesians 4:22–32; Colossians 3:5–17). He guides all of our steps toward the goal of our becoming more like Him.

Change means that we exchange things that were previously good for what is presently the best. Even good things, when out of season, can work against us. What was best in our lives when our children were growing up is no longer useful to us. My lifestyle when I was going through chemotherapy is no longer totally applicable. I have to live in what is necessary for this day and this season.

I have experienced much change in the past year. My idea of "getting back to life" is not what I had thought. What I considered to be normal before cancer is no longer possible. I am a different person, and I require a new way of life. Establishing a new way of life takes energy and focus, as well as determination, patience, and discipline. My patience and determination have grown but are still not perfected, so I continue to pray for God to grow His character in me.

As we change, we don't forget the principles that once took our entire focus, but we build on those principles, and they expand to become relevant to our present lives and needs.

There are some areas where we must constantly be changing. For example, we are to grow in love. Love, like God who is love (1 John 4:8), does not change. Love is constant in its nature, but *the more we understand and receive God's love, it becomes an agent for change in our hearts and lives.*

Discipline is another area in which we must be constantly growing. The boundaries of our lives change as we acquire discipline. Though discipline is a constant principle, the particulars change according to our present season of life.

It is especially interesting to see the issue of change and growth in our puppy. We were gone for two weeks, and he was with our friends who took good care of him. However, now that he is home, we must reestablish his boundaries. Because he is older and has had different experiences at our friends' house, he is attempting to stretch his boundaries at home. And he has been in some major trouble the past few days. He has been the "only child" for two weeks, and forgot that at home he has to share life with the cat. And when he chases her, she doesn't hesitate to use her claws on him. Our friends have a fenced yard where he was free to run in safety. When he got home, he decided to wander onto our country road where he can get hurt, so he has been in "time out." He is learning discipline according to the present situation. And sometimes, he doesn't like the boundaries we set. He especially does not like the consequences he experiences when he exceeds his boundaries.

God's changes in our lives are always for our good, and life is much more peaceful when we embrace His work rather than resist it. If we will look for His hand and His character, we will find ourselves being grateful for situations that would otherwise cause us to grumble and complain.

Because Charlie and I want to protect our puppy from harm, we discipline him when he gets in dangerous situations. So much more, God loves us, knows the possibilities, and He disciplines us to keep us safe and to bring us into a deeper experience of His abundant life. His discipline is *proof of His love* and care for us (Hebrews 12:5–11).

As Charlie and I transition back into a routine, we are different people than we were when we left for Japan. The presence of God has impacted our lives.

Tuesday, November 4 —
Trusting God with the Unknowns of the Future

One of the most special and unexpected things that happened in Japan was that, as I shared what God has done while I underwent cancer treatment, the doors seemed to open even more for me to minister to and share with people. I told the ladies at a women's meeting that, during this experience, I rediscovered truths about God that I have taught for the past 25 years.

About 18 months ago, the Lord challenged me with ideas about the future of our nation. As He listed the possibilities of dramatic things that could happen, He asked how I would respond. Would I respond with joy and trust Him, or would I react with fear and anxiety? Honestly, His questions brought me to my knees, and I confessed that I had a long way to go before I could trust the Lord in certain situations.

And then came January and a diagnosis of cancer. The trust issue became very personal. The Lord has continually challenged me this year to trust and submit every area of my life and health to Him. I know what is right, but I have still struggled to walk according to His will. Struggling is not necessarily wrong or a sin. But I know that His Spirit must be victorious in every outcome. I will not give up until I completely trust in Him.

I know people who are living in fear and anxiety — from a variety of issues in their lives. Yet, no matter what the focus of the fears, the question remains, "Will we trust God?" Fear looks at the present and projects the "what if's" into the future. I am not saying that planning or setting goals is wrong. We need to prayerfully set goals for our future. But no matter what our situation, the answer is to trust the Lord, because He alone knows the future.

Years ago, friends taught us a song that said, ". . . when all things that surround become shadows in the light of You . . .".[35] In the past year, I have found that when I put my eyes on the Lord — when I focus on and put my faith in Him — the situations of the world become like shadows in the background, and the majesty and character of God become increasingly more clear.

When I put my trust in Him rather than in the circumstances, I experience His peace. Jesus told us that *we will* have tribulation as long as we live in the world. But He added that we are to be of good cheer. We are not to allow our hearts to be troubled or in turmoil, but we are to be at peace because He has overcome the world.

I have told you these things so that in Me you may have [perfect] peace and confidence. In the world you have tribulation and trials and distress and frustration; but be of good cheer [take courage; be confident, certain, undaunted]! For I have overcome the world. [I have deprived it of power to harm you and have conquered it for you.] (John 16:33 AMP).

We are to trust Him with our personal situations as well as with national and world issues. As I write this, we do not know what the future will hold for our nation. But we are called to put our trust in the Lord and rejoice in Him in all things.

In the coming presidential election, if our preferred candidate does not win, will we trust that God is bigger than any situation and confidently know that He can perform His Word and His promises will not fail? If our preferred candidate does win, will we trust the Lord and realize that we are not to put our confidence and hope in people, governments, policies, economies, or institutions?

Our lives can only be healed when we trust God to work in and through us. In the same way, if our nation is to be healed, it will only come when those who are called by His name trust Him above all earthly institutions. We are to humble ourselves, pray, turn from our evil ways, and seek Him above all, surrendering all things in life to His divine and sovereign hand (2 Chronicles 7:14).

God kept asking me if I could trust Him to be more powerful than cancer, pain, or chemicals, as well as self-focus, doubt, and fear. And I can testify that *His presence is more powerful than anything I have ever experienced*. If we will turn to Him and trust Him to be God, He will do amazing things and set us free. I have seen that in the past year. I expect to see Him work powerfully even more in the coming years.

Sunday, November 9 — Living a "Normal" Life

This week has been as close to normal as I have had in months. It has been a good week. I even began to exercise again at the fitness center. As I exercise more regularly, I believe it will help build my strength. I am dieting as well, wanting to get rid of the weight I gained during chemotherapy. The only side effects I am having so far from the follow-up treatment is that often my body, especially my joints, aches when I move.

After I make myself move around, the pain decreases. Also, I don't sleep much at night, though that may not be a result of the medication. I will return to the oncologist in a few weeks for a checkup.

Earlier this week, I had blood tests, and my blood count was normal. On Tuesday afternoon, the surgeon will finally remove my port. I am so ready! Any infusions I have from now on will be through the veins in my arm, which is easier for me. I will then have only one more minor surgery, but that will probably not be for a while.

Yesterday I spent time with my grandchildren. It was fun to be together again with the family doing normal activities.

This time of the year, I begin to think about the holidays. Getting ready this year will be a little easier because the Christmas tree is still up! (I may be the only person who has to dust my Christmas tree!) The holiday season always helps prepare my heart for the coming year.

This has been an extraordinary year, but I am grateful that I don't have to go through the year of events again! And I don't want to spend the future reliving the past. I am looking forward to starting a new year with all the promise the future holds. I plan to move forward, focusing with hope and gratitude on the new things that God wants to do in my life.

In the coming year, I want to build on the good things God has done this year, and He still has almost two months of "building" to do before this year ends.

Tuesday, November 12 — Knowing the Basis of Our Identity

We each have an identity. We are known by certain things here on earth. Charlie says people most often identify themselves by what they do, who they know, or what they own. We each see ourselves one way, and those around us see us with their own perspectives. Most of my life, I have been known as Charlie's wife and Carie and Christie's mother, then a mother-in-law, and now "Grammy." Each of these represents precious relationships. Recently, I have been my doctors' patient.

Sometimes we identify people according to their circumstances, and a diagnosis of cancer can overshadow everything in a person's life. The past year, many seemed to see me primarily as a cancer patient. I was grateful that they were aware of what I was experiencing, and it was a huge blessing when I knew they were praying. Yet, I considered cancer as an issue to deal with, not my identity. I never referred to "my cancer." I felt that cancer was an invasion into my life and body, but I never wanted to own it. I have continued to think of myself as a healthy person who has had cancer. I have spent the year trying to live as normal a life as possible, within the limitations. I have wanted to accomplish things with the energy I had, rather than thinking of myself as a sick person who could do nothing. I knew if I allowed myself, I could use sickness as an excuse to avoid doing certain things. I didn't want to go there! Before my first surgery, the anesthesiologist asked me a long list of questions about my health. He ended by saying, "You are actually a very healthy person." I laughed and said, "Yes, other than having cancer, I am very healthy!" He responded by saying they were getting ready to remove the cancer.

I have heard people identify themselves as "cancer survivors." The fact is, I have survived this year, though I have survived because of the Lord's amazing grace and the people He brought into my life to help me heal. I often remind myself of His desire that I prosper and be in good health in both my body and my soul (3 John 2). My deepest desire is to have a soul that prospers in spiritual issues and then to enjoy the results.

As I have been asking the Lord for vision, He has been teaching me how to see myself as He sees me. I have learned that my true identity is not based on

- my body or my outward appearance, my hair, my physical condition;

- my health;

- my past;

- the works of my hands; or

- my education or profession.

The real "me" is the inner person, the "character" of the one who lives inside my human shell; I am who God says I am. The challenge is to know what God says about me and then, by faith, to agree with Him. Then I can walk more confidently as a child of God.

Here are just a few things God says we are. I am

- His witness and servant (Isaiah 43:10);

- one who has sinned and fallen short of God's glory, yet is justified by the grace of Jesus Christ (Romans 3:23-24);

- adopted by God, accepted, redeemed, forgiven of sins (Ephesians 1:3-14);

- one who has hope, peace, access to grace by faith, and I have the love of God in my heart (Romans 5:1-5);

- victorious (1 Corinthians 15:57);

- no longer a slave, but a child of God with full inheritance (Galatians 4:6-7);

- chosen, holy, and without blame, having every spiritual blessing in Christ (Ephesians 1:3-14);

- sealed with the Holy Spirit of promise (Ephesians 1:3-14);

- a citizen of the household of God who is being joined together with others to be a holy temple in the Lord — a dwelling place of God's Spirit (Ephesians 2:19-22);

- a citizen of heaven (Philippians 3:20);

- delivered from darkness and transferred into the Kingdom of the Son of God (Colossians 1:13-14); and

- a member of a chosen generation, a royal priesthood, a holy nation, His own special people, called out of darkness into His marvelous light, who has obtained mercy (1 Peter 2:9-10).

If I have any desire for how I am remembered, I want to be known as a faithful servant of the Almighty God and a recipient of His mercy and grace. Truly, life is about Him and all He does in and through our lives. I want to represent Him to the world.

I, like many of you, have walked through tribulation, but I have not walked alone. I am surrounded by the presence of a loving God and by His loving people who have encouraged me and prayed for me. That has made a difference, not only in my situation this past year but in who I am today.

Thank you for your prayers this week. All went well yesterday. I finally saw the doctor about 5 p.m., and she was finished with the surgery in 30 minutes. Charlie called it my "coming-out party." No more port! Yeah! I have a huge patch and stitches and some soreness. I am filled with gratitude to be this far along in the healing process.

Saturday, November 16 — Witnessing Restoration

In the middle of the night, I awoke with pain under my right arm. It went away, and I went back to sleep. I didn't think about it again until morning, when I had another pain in the same place. Then I realized, "I feel pain!" That was exciting, because that part of my arm has been numb since early March when I had the second surgery to remove lymph nodes. I had been told that the feeling might never return, but the pain may mean that the nerves have begun to repair themselves and start working again. So I have feeling! YEAH!

Tuesday, November 18 — Maintaining My Spiritual Life

I like our house to be clean and in order. However, it has become cluttered and dirty because I have not regularly cleaned cabinets and drawers. Normally, when I see something dirty, I immediately clean it, but I have not routinely maintained our home during the past year. Now I find myself feeling overwhelmed with things that need attention. I am trying to walk in peace, to pace myself, and to be satisfied to accomplish things as my energy allows.

Our spiritual lives can be like that. When we don't maintain our lives, we can become overwhelmed. When I don't daily focus on my relationship with the Lord, read the Bible, pray, and listen to what God has to say, I soon feel far away from Him. Then my mind tells me how difficult and time consuming it will be to get where I need to be.

However, my relationship with Him isn't that way. I need only to stop, ask the Lord to forgive me, and turn toward Him, simply returning to my daily routine of seeking Him again. The road back to the Lord is not long but is usually 180°. We have to turn and go toward Him rather than away from Him.

I have found that it is much more blessed to maintain my relationship with Him on a regular basis, rather than have to go back and try to catch up, patch, repent, and return to the place of peace where He wants me to be.

God's grace is truly amazing. *He doesn't make it difficult for us to be in His presence*. He wants us to be in relationship with Him and walk in His will. But we must do our part. He is constantly pursuing us and drawing us to Himself, but will not force Himself on us. And it is so easy for things of the world, the urgency of life, the busyness of our schedules to distract us and draw us *from* Him, *into* ourselves, and *toward* the world. But when we turn our eyes again on Him, we find He is right there waiting for us.

Recently, the Lord has challenged me with a Scripture I memorized years ago, "Do not love the world nor the things in the world. If anyone loves the world, the love of the Father is not in him" (1 John 2:15 NASB). This verse has pierced my heart lately, as I have recognized things of the world that I hold onto tightly. When I desire things, those things quickly replace or at least cloud my love for the Lord. Nothing is worth that price.

Months ago, when I realized that I was going to lose my hair, that loss seemed monumental. But now, I realize that what I consider physical necessities are small compared to the love of God. It isn't that He does not care about my feelings, but, through losing my hair, I discovered something far greater — *love doesn't rely on my outward appearance*! How extraordinary to know that who I am is not based on my outer shell but on my inner person. And honestly, the older I get and the more I face new physical limitations that come with age, the more I need to know that my value depends on spiritual things — on the love of the Father — and not on the things of the world . . . even my physical body.

The passage in 1 John goes on to say, "For all that is in the world, the lust of the flesh and the lust of the eyes and the boastful pride of life, is not from the Father, but is from the world. The world is passing away, and also its lusts; but the one who does the will of God lives forever" (1 John 2:16–17 NASB). Unless we have discernment, we can be drawn away from God by the world. The things of the world have no lasting value and bring little satisfaction. If we ask, His Spirit within us will show us anything that we value more than God.

So I am focusing on things of eternal value, realizing today's portion may not be spectacular or huge but will most likely be accomplished as I am faithful in the menial and as I seek first the Kingdom of God and His righteousness.

Thank You, Lord, for allowing us to know and serve You. Thank You for showing us glimpses of the beauty of the King and the Kingdom of God. The best the world can offer pales in comparison to You. Forgive us when we settle for the things of the world that are decaying and passing away. Thank You that You do not give up on us, but You keep drawing us to Yourself. You truly are Wonderful to love us frail humans with such great love.

Thursday, November 20 — Giving Thanks Is Primarily an Attitude

On Tuesday morning, I had an appointment with the surgeon for a checkup, to ensure that I am healing properly. Her assistant told me I was "perfect." I knew she was saying I was healing just as I should and, though I was not surprised, this *is* good news. I have an appointment tomorrow morning to have another surgical procedure. This procedure is more extensive than the one last week, but it is the finale. I told the surgeon I had to be healed in time to fix turkey and dressing for Thanksgiving next week.

Today, as Charlie and I were shopping for groceries, I got into a conversation with another shopper. She has been diagnosed with cancer twice and goes to the same surgeon and oncologist who have treated me. We talked for 30 minutes, and I had an opportunity to share with her some of the good things God has done for me in the past year. She talked about how her life and priorities changed and her appreciation of life increased.

I am amazed at how many things we become grateful for when times are tough. Thanksgiving is more than a day set apart; it is an attitude and daily lifestyle. Giving thanks and praise are great weapons against discouragement, doubt, fear, and other attitudes that we often let creep into our hearts. Every day, we can rejoice in God and all the good gifts He has given to us (James 1:17).

Saturday, November 22 — Seeing God Answer Prayers

All went well with the final surgical procedure. I was awake during the procedure (not my preference). The surgeon removed a mass of flesh on the side that was still partially numb. As a result of the numbness, I have had little pain. I slept well last night, and I am resting this weekend. I have tackled a few small projects in preparation for Thanksgiving, but I stop often to rest.

I hope each of you are also encouraged and see how God has heard and abundantly answered *your* prayers this year. Many of you have cried and laughed with me and now are rejoicing with me. I love you for being part of my life, and I love the Lord even more for placing each of you as a gift in my life. May He pour out His blessings of peace and joy on you this day, no matter what the situations are in your life, and may you experience His great faithfulness.

❦ GUEST

I am fascinated by the step-by-step process we must follow as the Holy Spirit brings us into God's plans. You are right: the process is important. Otherwise, we miss so much of what could have been.

Lately, I have found Scriptures in Matthew 6 and Luke 12 before me — about not being anxious about our lives. What excellent analogies Jesus gave about birds and flowers and the way they are adorned and provided for with no hint of worry. We have much to learn about the simple things of life and God's unchanging nature of love and faithfulness.

I believe one of the strongest tactics the enemy of our souls uses is busyness. It is wisdom to slow down and gaze upon God.

With a thankful heart for God's goodness and mercy in your healing,

Dianna

Monday, December 1 — Learning Valuable Principles by Which to Live

Last December, a friend gave me a large set of decorative gold keys. She said they represented keys that God was going to give me that would be significant insights and revelation of His Word and His character, principles that God wanted to build into my life for the future. I have recognized some of the keys that God gave to me this past year. Most of the "keys" are not new principles but are increased understanding that God has worked into my life.

The first principle that He spoke soon after the New Year was that I was not to be afraid. "Fear not, for I am with you" (Isaiah 41:10a ESV), and "Even though I walk through the valley of the shadow of death, I will fear no evil, for you are with me . . ." (Psalm 23:4a). No matter what happens in my personal life, health, finances, or in government and world economies, God knows all and I can trust Him and not be afraid. He is with me, and His presence makes the difference.

The second principle was also simple, yet profound. "In every thing give thanks: for this is the will of God in Christ Jesus concerning you . . ." (1 Thessalonians 5:18 KJV). God never said to give thanks *for* everything, but *in* everything. I find it impossible to be thankful *for* terrorists, thieves, abuse, disease, and other evils in the world. But, even in the midst of challenging circumstances, we can find things for which we can rejoice.

Thanksgiving Day has always been special. When I was growing up, football was the big family event on Thanksgiving Day. However, as I have grown older, my focus has changed. This year, I give thanks for things with eternal value. Life and relationships top that list.

I was reminded of something that happened years ago when we lived in the Washington, D.C. area. Each day, Charlie walked several blocks from our house to the bus stop and caught the bus to the Pentagon. One day when he was walking home, a young neighbor boy said, "Mister, your house caught on fire and burned down today." Charlie commented that he didn't think that was very funny. The young boy said he was not joking and that there was a fire in the next block on the left and it burned up the house. Charlie's slow-at-the-end-of-a-long-day pace immediately quickened. And between that conversation and the time he arrived at home, he reconciled that if the girls and I were alive and not hurt, nothing else mattered. When he got home, he discovered that it was the house next door that burned and not ours, but in his heart, he had settled the matter, knowing that family — not things — were most important. That night as we prayed for our neighbor and for what we could do to help her, we were very aware of the gift of family, safety, and health.

I am increasingly aware of the necessity of holding "things" loosely and holding tight to relationships. The privilege of fellowship with God and time with family and friends are not things I take for granted.

I pray that each of you had a wonderful Thanksgiving Day, and may the nearness of His presence make the difference in your life this and every day.

As I grow more aware of God's goodness and His blessings around me, I sometimes feel sad that my awareness and acknowledgment of His blessings seem minuscule compared to what He deserves. I have thought that "Every day should be Thanksgiving" because of all our daily blessings. But my human nature still wants to complain in conditions that most of the world would be so grateful to live in.

I appreciate your "keys" — giving thanks and not being afraid — because they speak to me about where I am and where I want to more fully move. I have to keep learning them and being reminded.

As this year closes and I look ahead with uncertainty, I keep reminding myself that fear comes when I am not focused on God and His Word. May our lives be enveloped in God's presence — He is enough! To say otherwise would be to unrighteously join ourselves to the things of this world.

Love always,
Dianna

Monday, December 8 — Dealing with Emotions

At the beginning of this journey, a friend told me I would have to fight the battle in three areas — the physical, the spiritual, and the emotional. I knew at that time the spiritual battle was the most familiar and where I am most experienced and effective. Much of the physical battle was left to the doctors, and I continue to follow their instructions. The pain was not as much a battle as was how I dealt with the pain, and the Lord was faithful to allow me to have minimal pain compared to what I knew was possible. He brought me through each day, each challenge, each trial. I have come to love and appreciate the word, "through." Psalm 23 says, "Yea, though I walk through the valley of the shadow of death, I will fear no evil: for You are with me" (v. 4a NKJV). We all go through difficult situations, and God is able to bring us through anything — even through death to resurrected life.

The emotional battle was the one for which I was least prepared. But I have learned a few things about emotions in the past year.

We are emotional beings. God made us in His image and likeness, and He is emotional. He

- laughs (Psalm 37:13);

- weeps (John 11:35; Luke 19:42);

- rejoices (Zephaniah 3:17 — I especially love this Scripture, and am amazed that He rejoices over me with singing.); and

- grows angry (Psalm 7:11; Isaiah 64:5; Hebrews 3:10).

Our culture often teaches us to deny our emotions. Women are considered "emotional beings" and are allowed to cry, while men are considered weak if they show any emotion. We forget that the most common emotion is anger. Men and women are both very capable of getting angry. And Scripture does not tell us *not* to be angry but that in our anger we are not to sin (Ephesians 4:26), and to deal with our anger quickly so as not to give the devil a foothold (Ephesians 4:27).

I remember the love and respect I felt for my husband the first time I saw him cry. He cried when my mother died shortly after we were married. But that was not the last time I saw him weep. I have seen him cry out of sadness, frustration, and joy — like when our daughters were born. Also, he has cried when the strong and loving presence of the Lord was touching his heart.

Years ago, when I was choir director in our church, the choir sang a song that really ministered to my heart. It was beautiful, and my tears flowed as the Spirit used the song to encourage me. After the church service was over, someone came and asked if Charlie and I were having problems in our marriage! I suspect she thought, as many do, that if you cry, something bad is happening. For sure, we sometimes cry because of pain or injustice, but sometimes we cry out of rejoicing.

Tears are sometimes very revealing of what is in our heart. If we cannot cry, we may be hard-hearted, bitter, or struggling with emotional pain that needs to be healed. I have had people cry with me and rejoice and laugh with me in the past year. What a precious gift, as their hearts were soft and were filled with compassion for me and my circumstances.

At the same time, I am aware that our tears can be used to manipulate others. That was a tactic I used early in our marriage. I am thankful to have grown beyond that in my life.

I continue to learn more about the "emotional battle" that comes with the diagnosis and treatment of cancer.

To keep our emotions buried is not healthy. We must learn to righteously deal with them and to use them as a gauge for what is going on in our lives. We must be able to look at ourselves honestly and confess how we are feeling.

Aiming our emotions at other people, like a weapon, is not healthy for anyone and is not what God intended. *We need to take responsibility for our own emotions rather than blaming them on other people or situations.* Rather than saying, "You make me so mad," we should admit, "When you do that, I get angry."

When our emotions, like the rest of our lives, are not under the control of the Holy Spirit, we are in danger of losing the battle. Emotions can be destructive if they are not surrendered to the Holy Spirit, and if they control our attitudes, words, actions, and decisions.

Certainly in the condition of our economy and in the world situations today, we can admit, "I am worried," "I am stressed," or "I am angry." And God has told us in the Scriptures about how to deal with these feelings. He tells us not to be anxious but in every situation, with thanksgiving, we should bring our prayers and petitions to God (Philippians 4:6), who can do something about our situations and who can give us peace in the midst of our circumstances. Blaming institutions, nations, individuals, or even groups of people hurts us and keeps us from dealing with our own issues and responses.

We are living in times and situations that are challenging, and the answer is to turn to God and to trust Him. No matter what comes our way, He says His name is above all names, and He is King of Kings and Lord of Lords. Nothing exists that can overcome God's power and love. He is even stronger than our emotions. We don't have to be controlled by our emotions, but we can submit them to Him, and He will faithfully lead us and guide us.

Blessings to you as you prepare your heart for Christmas. As the wonderful carol says, "Joy to the world! The Lord is come; let earth receive her King. Let every heart prepare Him room, and heaven and nature sing . . .".[36]

I always look forward to the New Year. Every year for almost 30 years, the Lord has given us a word of direction that showed something of what He would do in and through us during the coming year. We can look back and see how God accomplished those words in our lives. We know He is saying several things for this year, and we are seeking Him for what they mean. This year, the Lord is going to use all I experienced last year as equipping for the future.

During the past six months, the Lord has repeatedly spoken to me about "vision." I want to see with His perspective, but too often, my spiritual sight is clouded by my own understanding, experience, and emotions. I am thankful that He is willing and able to give us wisdom so we can see as He does . . . if we will ask (James 1:5).

The past year was like getting corrected lenses. The journey — finding the tumor, walking through the diagnoses, learning the options and praying for wisdom, undergoing treatment, seeking the Lord and seeing Him answer prayer and work miracles, feeling the love of family and friends — has given me new focus. I see many things more clearly now; I respond to many things in life differently. This is not physical sight, but spiritual sight — seeing with my heart. My spiritual understanding has greatly increased, and I see people and situations in a new way.

I am thankful for the changes that have taken place in my life this year. It has been extraordinary, and I would not change all I have learned for anything. Now, I anticipate how the "change in vision" will impact the coming year. A new journey begins, and I pray it will be as rewarding as the past journey.

My most frequent prayer during the past year has been to remind Him, "Lord, you have to use this for my good" (Romans 8:28.) I'm not talking about "everything always works out for good no matter who we are or what we do." That is not truth. Most of His promises have conditions. God gives the promise for those who love Him and are called according to His purpose for them (Romans 8:28). If you are a child of God, then His promise is for you. If you have not given your life to Him, He is waiting and longing for you to do that. He loves you and desires a personal relationship with you; He wants you to walk in the blessings of His amazing promises. I pray that in the coming year, you will clearly see His hand move on your behalf, even in any difficult situation you may face.

I realize that though I have been proclaimed "cancer free," this journey is not over. Two weeks ago, the oncologist said he wants to do a PET scan to ensure that the cancer has not reoccurred in another part of my body. I was not fearful when he said that, but I was surprised, as I had never considered that I might have to go through this again. I am not expecting to, but no matter what the future brings, I am seeking to use every day to its fullest.

I continue to pray that God will enable me to "finish the race" of this life with zeal, passion, and purpose. I will die one day. Even Lazarus, who was raised from the dead (John 11), eventually died again. But I don't want to die before my time has been completed (Psalm 139:16), and I want every moment to count for eternity.

Life can change in a moment. The day I discovered the tumor, I knew my life would change. From that day on, I learned the process and discovered the details of how much and in what ways things would change. Even two weeks ago, the physical therapist gave me a list of things I must do in the future — changes that I must make for the rest of my life as a result of having cancer and surgery. In the future, I will realize more and more of what God did in my life during the past year — not only in healing me but also in building me up spiritually as I learned to lean on Him in deeper measure.

Change can come on a personal and individual level, but it can also come on a national and world level. Change can come suddenly or gradually. But in every case, we can have hope and we can pray, knowing that God continues to work on our behalf.

I have come to realize in a greater measure the power of the Word of God. His Word is not a magic wand that we wave over situations, but *it has creative power* as it did in "the beginning," when God's spoken word created the universe.

- God spoke the world into being (Genesis 1 — see what happened every time "God said").

- Jesus is "the Word of God" (John 1:1), and the Word became flesh and lived among us (John 1:14).

- Jesus is the revelation of God, who does not lie. He is the Truth (John 14:6). His Word is truth (John 17:17), and His Word is relevant to each of us and to each of our situations, if we will simply trust Him.

His Word has the power to heal, protect, and provide because His Word cannot be separated from who He is; He is the healer, protector and provider. Salvation is the process of becoming *one* with the living Word, Jesus. It is amazing that as we meditate on the written Scriptures, they reveal Him, and they also become personalized for our lives.

In Scripture, the English for "word" is given two meanings. The *logos* word is an expression of thought, and normally refers to the written Scriptures. The *rhema* word is when the Spirit of God highlights or quickens to us a particular passage, and we know it is the exact word needed for our specific and individual situation.

Vine's Expository New Testament Dictionary says,

> The significance of rhema (as distinct from logos) is exemplified in the injunction to take 'the sword of the Spirit, which is the word of God, (Eph. 6:17); here the reference is not to the whole Bible as such, but to the individual Scripture which the Spirit brings to our remembrance for use in time of need, a prerequisite being the regular storing of the mind with Scripture.[37]

God's Word is completely trustworthy and relevant to today and to the individual challenges of our lives. God knew that this time in our history and economy would come. And He is still able to perform His Word in our lives. God's Word has stood the test of time. Yet, for each of us, His Word must stand the test in our own lives.

God is so loving and powerful that even when the world around us seems to be crumbling, the Rock of Ages has not changed (Malachi 3:6). He is able to perform His Word in our lives, He is able to take care of us, and He is able to provide. He tells us not to worry or to lean on our own understanding but to acknowledge Him in all things and not to be wise in our own eyes (Proverbs 3:5–7). He says not to build our lives on "sand" but on the rock, which is Jesus (Matthew 7:24–27). And He tells us to "[cast] all your cares on him, because *he cares* for you" (1 Peter 5:7 LEB). He *wants* to take care of us, all the time.

Recently, I was praying for a friend, and as I prayed, I felt doubt and unbelief rise up in my heart. Inside, I did not believe God would do what I was asking for. I was not hopeful but was actually discouraged as I prayed. I asked the Lord to show me what to do. I wanted to pray in faith.

He said, "Stop praying the situation and pray *Me*!" I understood that, as I was praying, I was focused on the situation, which seemed hopeless. I was having difficulty praying and was not able to pray a faith-filled prayer. I began praying again with my focus on God and His ability. I prayed His Word into my friend's life. I prayed what I knew was true, because it was what God says, both about Himself and about my friend.

> "Thank You, Lord, that You love Your daughter so much that You suffered and died for her. And Father, You said, 'He who did not spare his own Son, but gave him up for us all—how will he not also, along with him, graciously give us all things?' (Romans 8:32). You will use this for her good because You promised (Romans 8:28). You do not break your promises. Lord, show her Your faithfulness. Thank You that You are completely faithful, no matter what our situations look like (2 Timothy 2:13). Thank You that You don't have any problems, but You can use all situations to demonstrate Your glory. Thank You for being all that my friend needs at this moment. Pour out Your grace and mercy on her life. I love You and thank You for who You are!"

When I finished praying, I *knew* God had heard my prayers and was already moving in a mighty way in my friend's life. How amazing is that? I did not see any changes in her situation for several months, and now I watch as the Lord continues to provide for her.

Prayer is not like shooting a gun into the air and hoping we will hit something. It is two-way communication in a personal relationship with the Creator and King of the universe, who has all power and all knowledge and who loves us with an everlasting love. Wow! What a privilege. It involves agreeing with the intercession Jesus and His Holy Spirit are constantly offering to the Father on our behalf (Romans 8:26-28, 34). I often think that much of prayer is for us. God knows what great things He wants to do. He just needs for us to link our faith with His will.

So, whatever you are facing this day—whatever changes have come into your life—God wants to help you. He has no problems but uses every situation to reveal His glory, His love, and His power to us. His grace is sufficient (2 Corinthians 12:9). I encourage you, in the midst of your challenging circumstances, to look to God and to trust Him to work mightily. Ask Him to prove His faithfulness to you. Surrender the situation to Him and acknowledge that He alone can solve it. Trust Him. He is God.

Mom, thank you for your words of wisdom. So frequently, I forget to pray "God" and instead pray my circumstances. I need to remember that God is in control and that, while He does not cause hardships, He will use them if we pray in His will.

Carie

Tuesday, August 4 — Celebrating One Year Later

Yesterday, I had an MRI. I had not had one since before my first surgery. I forgot how exhausting it is when I go to the hospital and they inject chemicals into my body! I sometimes think I am back to normal until I overload a day. Today, I must rest and allow my strength to rebuild.

I can hardly believe it has been an entire year since I had my last chemotherapy treatment. To look at me, no one would know that I had been through cancer and chemotherapy. My hair has grown back enough so that I just look like I have a short haircut. I have eyebrows, and my eyelashes are growing. I have lost 10 pounds, and most days my strength is good. I am thankful.

God has allowed me to meet people who are walking through cancer and chemotherapy and other challenging situations. I am more equipped to minister to these people because of what I experienced last year. My faith has grown tremendously since this process began 18 months ago.

I continue on the road to restoration, and am being patient. Healing and restoration don't always come as quickly as we might prefer. I am thankful to be this far along. Your prayers and encouragement have been instrumental in getting me here.

Friday, August 14 — Working in My Body and My Heart

Yesterday, I received a call from the surgeon saying that the result of the MRI is normal, and my oncologist called to say that the PET scan shows no cancer cells in my body. I rejoice in good reports.

I want to share one additional thing. The Lord showed me that what was going on in my physical body last year was a picture of what He was doing inside my heart. He was infusing His Spirit into me to combat attitudes that did not belong. His Spirit attacked and removed fears, lies I had believed for years, people-pleasing, and other things that had the potential to damage my soul, as cancer does to the body. I have recently realized that spiritually, mentally, and emotionally, I am healthier today than I have been in years or maybe ever in my life. God has worked on my physical health and my spiritual health. I will be eternally grateful for all the blessings that came out of last year.

I am aware that, as I have gained strength, I am more tempted to walk in my own strength rather than rely on the Lord as I did last year. I don't want to lose that new level of reliance on Him that I came to love and cherish so deeply.

❧ GUEST

Thank you for sharing your journey with all of us. I am comforted and encouraged by the evidence of God's grace and mercy as He has led you along this tough journey.

Recently a friend of mine here in Sacramento was diagnosed with breast cancer, and I referred her to your journal here on CaringBridge. I am praying for opportunities to "be there" for her in practical ways. A few women from our church are also interested in assisting with meals or going to her chemo sessions with her. What are some practical ways that others have ministered to you?

Kathy

Thursday, October 29 — Seeking Practical Ways to Minister

Dear Kathy,

Thank you for your encouragement and your question. I know your question comes from a heart of compassion, love, and service. I thank God for giving us a desire to make a difference.

Some of the following are from my experience and some come from friends walking through cancer. The information may reveal some potential areas of struggle for your friend and her family.

Pray

The first thing you can do is something you are already doing: *pray, pray, pray*. Prayers were invaluable to me. Many days I didn't have the strength to pray for myself, but I knew others were praying for me. I have heard people say they could "feel the prayers." It was true. I felt protected and could just "*be*" with Him.

Pray for your friend's caregivers. Sometimes, those who are closest, especially family, feel the most helpless. They definitely have their own struggles and often have to deal with their own fears. They can then feel guilty for their own struggles because they are not the person who is sick. A husband who desires to protect can have a difficult time dealing with the fact that he cannot change or fix the situation.

Pray for her family. Her children may have to deal with their own fears of getting cancer or of losing their Mom.

Provide Meals

Taking meals can be a blessing. Ask questions first: When would she like the meals? What kinds of foods does she like? Is there anything she cannot eat? Meals can especially be a blessing even if your friend cannot eat, because her family needs to be fed. Ask if the family members have allergies, or if her doctor has restricted her diet.

Many people sent us meals. However, Carie did all of the coordinating of meals. The food was delivered to her house and she delivered it to us. I knew I was not able to visit with people, so that was a protection of my strength.

Communicate Encouragement

Cards were a very special gift. I have a friend who sent me a card every week with an encouraging message. I still have them all, as the messages are timeless. The written responses on CaringBridge also brought life to me. I felt like I was running a race, and those on the sideline were cheering me on! Some were even running part of the way with me. I never felt "alone." Affirmation that God loves me and still has a good plan for my life was always something I loved hearing; I still do!

Another friend sent me flowers and plants regularly while I was going through chemotherapy. They always brightened up the house and encouraged me. Note that some people have allergies to certain plants, so it is best to ask rather than assume. You can send silk flower arrangements. I have enjoyed those and they don't have to be watered!

Listen

Much of the time I didn't have the energy to talk. But at times, I needed to verbally process what I was thinking and feeling. Knowing that I had someone I could call who would listen was comforting. I had friends who would cry with me and laugh with me. Listening is truly a gift of love.

Provide Normalcy

I wanted people to see me as Suzanne — a real person. At times, I needed to forget that I had cancer. I have a close friend who wanted people to come over and play board games or cards or watch a fun movie with her — to do something normal when she had the energy. My grandchildren were great fun during those times. I wanted to live life to the fullest when I had the energy. My life, goals, visions, and calling did not stop. My friend, like me, wanted conversation that did not focus on hospitals, sickness, and treatment. I laughed lots and enjoyed being with people who were free to laugh with me.

Offer to Help

I also appreciated when people asked if they could do anything for me. It showed me that they cared. Some people demonstrate love through doing things for you. I was thankful when they accepted a "no" answer, but I also was grateful to know they were available in case I did need a ride to the hospital, meals, or something in case of an emergency. Availability was a precious gift.

If your friend has to go to the hospital often, you can offer to take her and bring her home. I do not think I could have driven myself home after chemotherapy. Charlie normally took me, and sometimes he would stay with me during the treatment. Carie came to almost every treatment and would bring lunch. I always looked forward to seeing her and the children.

If your friend has small children, she may need childcare or help getting older children to or from school.

Charlie found a lady who would clean our house every two weeks. That was a huge blessing, as I did not have the energy to clean. However, some people cannot afford that. You might offer to help with cleaning or chores around the house. Also, there are organizations that provide house cleaning services for breast cancer patients.

Be Sensitive

Let your friend define her needs. If you need to, ask her what she needs, and keep the door of communication open. That is always better than assuming you know what she needs.

If she wants someone with her, knowing you, you will be there. If she needs to be alone, then I know you will have the sensitivity to sit back and wait. You have great sensitivity — I have always loved that about you. I have not often been a person who wants to be "left alone." Usually, the more the merrier. But when I went through surgery and chemotherapy, I withdrew, mostly because of my lack of energy and strength. When people were around, I felt compelled to focus on their needs, and it took more energy than I had. It kept me from resting.

I was never offended by "How are you doing?" I was always grateful when it came with a smile rather than a worried frown. I was grateful when I said "Fine" and people accepted that I was either not up to talking or that I actually was doing okay that day. I especially appreciated when they didn't press me for details. (See my journal entry for May 7.) I didn't want pity; I wanted love and compassion.

Ask about Additional Prayer Focuses

In the physical realm, the doctors gave me so much information that I was on overload. The books and pamphlets related every possible and extreme outcome, side effect, result. Not everyone is as easily overloaded as I was. Some have more medical knowledge than I have. Some need to know all the details and seek for it on the internet. But, I would read a few pages and be able to do nothing but cry; I couldn't process it all — mentally or emotionally. Carie went through the information and shared with me what I needed to know when I needed to know it. That was a huge relief. If you have any medical knowledge, you can offer to help in this area.

At the same time that I was trying to process all of the information, I was also working to keep my focus on God. Some days that seemed impossible.

The things I was reading were very negative, and I often grew discouraged and fearful. It was difficult to tune in to hear God's "still small voice."

I understand that doctors have to give this information to patients to legally protect themselves. Your friend may have to cope with feeling of overload from the information. It takes time and prayer to weed out all that is not of God and seek Him in the midst of this. I appreciated when people would help point me back to God and His faithfulness and love.

Draw Near to Your Friend

Often, people didn't know what to say to me, so they avoided me. I understood that. Sometimes, people would look at me and I could see fear in their eyes. It seems that facing me made them afraid of what could happen to them. I found myself wanting to assure them of God's presence, His love, and His power. Disease does not separate us from God.

Most of all, remember that you hear God. As you ask Him what you are to do, He will guide you, and it may be "none of the above." Your friend will have her own walk, her own needs, her own perspective in this journey. It probably will be totally different from mine. But God will lead you to do the right thing because your heart is in the right place. You are a person of genuine care and love, who demonstrates God's Spirit. That will shine through to your friend. Let her know how precious and valuable she is to you. Just be the caring person I know you to be. She is blessed to have a friend like you. That is what the Body of Christ is all about.

Again, thank you for asking. Your question helped me think through some things of the past year. It also reminded me, once again, of the many people who supported, helped, and blessed me in so many ways.

I will join you in praying for your friend.

References

[1] Yancey, P. (2006). *Prayer: Does it make any difference?* Grand Rapids, MI: Zondervan.

[2] Smith, B. (1989). No sugar apple pie. In *Protestant Women of the Chapel, Yokota AB, Japan [Cookbook]*. Olathe, KS: Cookbook Publishers, Inc.

[3] Van DeVenter, J.W. (1896). *I surrender all.* Public domain.

[4] Sheets, D. (2006). *Authority in prayer: Praying with power and purpose.* Bloomington, MN: Bethany House Publishers.

[5] Patterson, S. (2008, March 11). A global view of breast cancer: Middle-Eastern women surmount stigma, danger to share stories. *Dallas Morning News.* Retrieved from http://www.dallasnews.com/sharedcontent/ dws/fea/columnists/spatterson/stories/DNnh_patterson_0311liv.ART.State.Edition1. 4637bf9.html

[6] Alves, E. (1992). *The mighty warrior: A guide to effective prayer.* Bulverde, TX: Canopy Press.

[7] Wallis, A. (1986). *God's chosen fast: A spiritual and practical guide to fasting.* Ft. Washington, PA: Christian Literature Crusade.

[8] Smith, M. (1994). *I could sing of your love forever.* United Kingdom: Music UK.

[9] Spafford, H.G., & Bliss, P. P. (1876). *It is well with my soul.* Public domain.

[10] Chisholm, T. (1923). *Great is Thy faithfulness.* Public domain.

[11] Holloway, Terese. (2010). Seeds of Hope. *My destiny is Jesus.* Lake Mary, FL: Creation House.

[12] Forsake. (n.d.). *Encarta World English Dictionary.* Retrieved from http://encarta.msn.com/encnet/features/dictionary/DictionaryResults.aspx?lextype= 3&search=forsake

[13] Gungor, M., & Houghton, I. (2003). *Friend of God.* Mobile, AL: Integrity Music Inc.

[14] Petrarca, L. (2010, April 26). Eagle in a storm. *Bowl of inspiration: A heaping bowl of encouragement daily.* Retrieved from http://bowlofinspiration.blogspot.com/2010/04/eagle-in-storm.html

[15] Bannister, B., & Hudson, M. (1978). *Praise the Lord.* Nashville, TN: WordMusic, Inc.

[16] Dread. (n.d.). *Encyclopedia Britannica, Inc.* Retrieved from Dictionary.com website: http://dictionary.reference.com/browse/dread

[17] Vine, W.E., Unger, M.F., & White, W. (1996). "Hope." *Vine's complete expository dictionary of Old and New Testament words.* Nashville, TN: Thomas Nelson.

[18] Upton, J. (2007). *In Your presence.* Sydney, Australia: Hillsong Music.

[19] Cloud, H., & Townsend, J. (1992). *Boundaries: When to say YES, when to say NO, to take control of your life.* Grand Rapids, MI: Zondervan.

[20] Spafford, H.G., & Bliss, P. P. (1876). *It is well with my soul.* Public domain.

[21] Webster, N. (1828). Rest. *American dictionary of the English language.* New York, NY: S. Converse.

[22] Lakewood Church. (2004). *Glorify Your name.* Minato, Tokyo, Japan: Sony.

[23] Parish, F. (1999). *Honor: What love looks like.* Ventura, CA: Renew.

[24] Flint, A.J. (1996). He giveth more grace. In H. Gapriepy (Ed.), *Songs in the night.* Grand Rapids, MI: Eerdmans Publishing. Cited in Hughes, R.K. (1991). *Faith that works.* Wheaton, IL: Crossway Books.

[25] Beijing 2008. (2005). Humanity: John Stephen Akhwari—The greatest last place finish ever. Retrieved from http://en.beijing2008.cn/29/16/article212011629.shtml

[26] Webster, N. (1828). Bear (verb). *American dictionary of the English language.* New York, NY: S. Converse.

[27] American Cancer Society. (n.d.) *MoreBirthdays.com – American Cancer Society: Official sponsor of birthdays.* Retrieved from http://morebirthdays.com

[28] Vine, W.E., Unger, M.F., & White, W. (1996). Miracle. *Vine's complete expository dictionary of Old and New Testament words: With topical index.* Nashville, TN: T. Nelson.

[29] Browning, E.B., & Kaplan, C. (1978). *Aurora Leigh, and other poems* (1st ed.). London, UK: The Women's Press.

[30] Vine, W.E., & Fleming, M.A. (1996) poikilos. *An expository dictionary of New Testament words* (3rd ed.). Old Tappan, NJ: H. Revel Co.

[31] Hastings, J. (Ed.). (1989). *Hastings Bible dictionary* (abridged). Peabody, MA: Hendrickson Publishers.

[32] Webster, N. (1967). Infusion (verb). *Webster's Seventh New Collegiate Dictionary.* Springfield, MA: G. & C. Merriam Company.

[33] Vine, W.E., Unger, M.F., & White, W. (1996). Hope. *Vine's complete expository dictionary of Old and New Testament words: With topical index.* Nashville, TN: T. Nelson.

[34] ten Boom, C., Sherrill, J., & Sherrill, E. (1971). *The hiding place.* Old Tappan, NJ: Fleming H. Revell Company.

[35] Perrin, W., & Perrin, C. (1981). *When I look into Your holiness.* Mobile, AL: Integrity Music Inc.

[36] Watts, I. (1748). *Joy to the world! The Lord is come.* Public domain.

[37] Vine, W.E., Unger, M.F., & White, W. (1996). Rhema. *Vine's complete expository dictionary of Old and New Testament words: With topical index.* Nashville, TN: T. Nelson.

www.ingramcontent.com/pod-product-compliance
Lightning Source LLC
Chambersburg PA
CBHW051137020726
47501CB00005B/1551